How We Grieve

How We Grieve

Relearning the World

REVISED EDITION

Thomas Attig

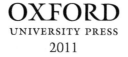

OXFORD

UNIVERSITY PRESS

2011

OXFORD

UNIVERSITY PRESS

Oxford University Press
Oxford New York
Athens Auckland Bangkok Bombay
Calcutta Cape Town Dar es Salaam New Delhi
Florence Hong Kong Istanbul Karachi
Kuala Lumpur Madras Madrid Melbourne
Mexico City Nairobi Paris Singapore
Taipei Tokyo Toronto
and associated companies in Berlin Ibadan

Copyright © 1996, 2011 by Oxford University Press, Inc.

Published by Oxford University Press, Inc.,
198 Madison Avenue, New York, New York 10016

Oxford is a registered trademark of Oxford University Press

Library of Congress Cataloging-in-Publication Data
Attig, Thomas, 1945–
How we grieve : relearning the world /
Thomas Attig. — rev. ed.
p. cm.
Includes bibliographical references and index
ISBN 978-0-19-539769-7 (pbk. : alk. paper)
1. Bereavement—Psychological aspects.
2. Bereavement—Psychological aspects—Case studies.
3. Grief. 4. Grief—Case studies.
5. Death—Psychological aspects.
6. Loss (Psychology)—I. Title.
BF575.G7A79 2010
155.9'37—dc22
2010022373

Printed in the United States of America
on acid-free paper

For my children, Julie, Sheryl, and Dan.
May these reflections prove helpful one day.

Preface to the Revised Edition

Nearly fifteen years have passed since the first edition of *How We Grieve: Relearning the World* appeared. Since then I've expanded and deepened my thinking about the central ideas in the book. In part in response to work on related topics by others in the field. And in part as I have found vocabulary and come to insights that enable me to appreciate better the interpretive power of thinking of grieving as relearning the world. I share my expanded reflections in chapter-by-chapter commentary in the extensive "Introduction" to this revised edition.

I refer to and discuss other publications in which I have explored critically the implications of the phenomenology of grieving as relearning the world for central concerns in the field. Those writings are my best attempts to contribute constructively to discussions of complicated grief, disenfranchised grief, loss of the assumptive world, meaning-making in grief, continuing bonds, anticipatory grieving, grief and existential suffering in children, and respecting the spirituality of the bereaved.

I also offer commentary on several other issues in contemporary discussion. These include relief grief, the effectiveness of grief counseling, limitations of and an appropriate agenda for research in the field, efforts to develop a grief category for inclusion in the DSM, the five-stage theory of grief, the task model of grieving, the dual-process model of grieving, empathic failure, narrative ethics and respecting individuality, shifting emphasis on emotive and cognitive aspects of grieving, resilience, and closure.

I have come to appreciate the important distinction between *grief reaction* and *grieving response*. We relearn the world in grief reactions as we passively take in the realities of change in our world that bereavement entails, including the loss of wholeness and sorrow that come over us. And we relearn the world in grieving response as we actively come to terms with these changes in our world and reengage in the fullness of life. I stress grieving response in the book because other treatments of grieving either neglect it altogether or inadequately describe the labors of grieving.

I have also come to appreciate the nature and value of the emotional aspects of grief reaction. Emotions grip us until we give them the attention they deserve. They can teach us about our selves and what we need for survival and reengagement in the world. I describe sorrow-friendly practices (varieties of grieving response) we can use to actively engage with and learn from our grief reactions.

I correct a major misinterpretation of relearning the world as primarily a cognitive process. Rather than being a matter of *learning that* the world is different in the aftermath of loss, it is one of *learning how to be and act* in a world transformed by loss. Relearning the world requires changes in the patterns of needs, wants, emotions, motivations, interests, behaviors, habits, dispositions, interactions, expectations, and hopes that shape our caring engagement with the world, not just our ways of thinking about or narrating it.

I have a clearer understanding of the labors of grieving response that together enable us to relearn the world. We learn to carry the pain of missing the one we grieve, return home to and trust what remains of the familiar, stretch into the inevitably new in our daily life patterns and next chapters of our life stories, and learn to love in separation. We do much straightforwardly, without thinking. We self-consciously solve problems. We address and complete tasks. We undertake life-long projects of modifying our understandings, emotions, behaviors, and relationships. And we engage with the mysteries of finiteness, change, life, love, suffering, and death.

I have come to use a vocabulary of *ego, soul,* and *spirit* to flesh out my understanding of the nature of the self as it is embodied in a web of caring engagements in the world. It enables me to identify the soul and spirit as the deep forces within us that weave the webs of our daily life patterns and reweave them continuously into our life stories. It allows me to describe how the sorrow that comes over us in grief reaction includes not only the helplessness of our ego but also the homesickness of our soul and the fear and despair of our spirit. And it enables me to characterize the labors of relearning the world in terms of the distinctive reengagements of these three life-shaping forces in the world of our experience.

And I have come to appreciate more fully how learning to love in separation is the pivotal challenge in relearning the world. The world we relearn is filled with painful reminders of the separation, in our physical and social surroundings, and within our selves. We learn to carry the pain as we reach past it to embrace cherished memories and legacies the world also holds. This is the hope that enables us to transcend our suffering and relearn the world in life-affirming ways.

I am grateful to those whose works and thinking continue to stimulate, and sometimes provoke, my thinking, including Bill Worden, Ken Doka, Miriam Greenspan, Arthur Frank, Rita Charon, Bob Neimeyer, Jack Jordan, Dale Larson, Jeff Kaufman, Dennis Klass, Phyllis Silverman, Colin Parkes, Terrie Rando, Elisabeth Kubler-Ross, David Kessler, Holly Priggerson, Margaret Stroebe, Henk Schut, Irwin Sandler, and George Bonannos.

I also highly value the abiding support and enthusiasm for my work from colleagues and friends, including Mal and Di McKissock, Paul Rosenblatt, David Balk, David Meagher, Darcy Harris, Doug Daher, and Nancy Hogan.

And I would be especially remiss if I did not acknowledge those who have supported me in the preparation of this new edition, including Joan Bossert (my Oxford editor), Betty Davies (my wife and best critic), and Don Scherer (my dear friend and fellow applied philosopher).

Thomas Attig
Victoria, British Columbia

Preface to the First Edition

Edvard Munch's painting "The Death Chamber" depicts a sickroom moments after someone has died. It is the scene of his young sister's death years earlier, but the focus falls not on the deceased but rather on the survivors. The furnishings are sparse, with only a bed, two chairs, and a small portrait on the wall in view. Six persons are captured at the moment they absorb the first impact of the loss. A young man at the left rear faces away from the bed, leaning his hand on the wall with his head bent downward. A bearded elderly gentleman in the right center rear, next to the bed and behind a chair that holds an obscure figure, faces front with his hands folded in prayer. A middle-aged woman at the right rear stands with a featureless face bent down, bracing herself on that same chair. A young woman is seated in profile at the center front with her head bowed and her hands folded in her lap. Behind her and slightly to the left, another young woman stands and stares forlornly toward the front with her hands folded in front of her. Another young man stands behind with his back to the two young women and stares blankly toward the rear of the room.

Although the room is filled with people, it seems not at all crowded. Each figure is very much alone in his or her experience of what has just happened. Each is bereaved—deprived of the presence of the one with whom he or she had shared life but a few moments before. No one speaks. No one faces, much less approaches, another.

None touch or embrace. Each is stunned and still, frozen in place and lifeless. Each is withdrawn and vulnerable, reacting in isolation. Each recoils from the death and from the changed reality he or she now confronts. Each is suspended between the world as it was and the world as it is now, transformed utterly by the death. The absence of the one they love is palpable. Each seems at a loss as to what to do or say and how to go on from here, and especially at a loss as to what to do with the feelings he or she still has for the one who has died. None appears ready to leave the room, to face the world and life without the deceased. Yet that is precisely what each must do. For now, the death chamber is both the scene of the event that has changed the world as each experiences it and a quiet refuge from the challenges that a new world presents to each. Fortunately, although no one can grieve for another, when they leave the room, none will grieve alone. They will face the world together with fellow survivors and, in interaction with them, build new patterns of living in the absence of the deceased.

Few who have ever lost another can help being moved by Munch's treatment of the first moments after a loss. Bereavement, even when expected, leaves indelible memories and defines some of the most important turning points in our lives. We absorb the impacts of loss within our unique life circumstances and as the individuals we are. Each of us experiences the world in a way that is uniquely our own; within our worlds of experience we learn to feel, behave, think, expect, and hope as if those we care about will continue to live. When someone in our world dies, we remain postured in that world as we were before the death, but we can no longer sustain that posture. We are challenged to learn new ways of feeling, behaving, thinking, expecting, and hoping in the aftermath of the loss. As we learn these things, we cope. Grieving, by definition, is just such coping with the challenges that bereavement presents. Grieving is what we do in response to what happens to us in bereavement.

This book contains one philosopher's reflections on grieving as the centrally important human experience it is. It grows out of some twenty years of teaching and writing about death and dying, grief and bereavement. The teaching and writing, in turn, are rooted in at least that many years of careful listening to the stories of persons who, like those depicted in Munch's lithograph, have lost someone dear to them and struggled with how to go on living without the deceased. The book is written for all those who, with me, wonder what going on without the deceased involves—those who grieve, as well as the families, friends, members of support groups, and professionals who wonder how to support and comfort them. It is a book for those with theoretical and professional interests in bereavement and grieving, but it is written with the intention of reaching the broad audience I have just described.

In Chapter 1 I maintain that the point of thinking about grieving is to allow us to understand better the experiences of individuals who are grieving and to use that understanding to support and comfort them as they grieve. And, I clarify my intentions to provide the general understanding from others and of themselves in grief, respect for individuality, means of addressing helplessness, and guidance for caregivers that I believe persons seek when they turn to books on grieving. In Chapter 2 I survey common strands of current thinking, including stage/phase, medical, and task-based views of grieving. I criticize the stage/phase and the medical views as inadequate, refine the task-based view, and argue that it promises the most of what persons seek in understanding grieving and what caregiving requires. In Chapter 3 I show that respect for individuals as they grieve requires both that we not interfere in their grieving or exacerbate their vulnerability and that we facilitate their return to flourishing and full community with fellow survivors. In Chapter 4 I develop the central idea of grieving as a process of relearning the world that requires that we relearn physical surroundings and find a new place within them, relearn our relationships with others, including fellow survivors, the deceased, and (for some of us) God, and relearn ourselves, that is, our ways of being who we are. In Chapter 5 I provide a detailed description of how we suffer in the aftermath of loss and how we relearn our selves as we adjust our daily life patterns, redirect the stories of our lives, and establish new patterns of connection with the world. In Chapter 6 I show how it is possible and desirable to think of grieving as, in part, our making the transition from loving persons who are present to loving them in their absence.

Bowling Green, Ohio T.A.

Acknowledgments

Special thanks are due all the students in my death and dying classes and in my workshops on grief and bereavement, guest speakers in my classes, audience members for my presentations, and clients whom I have served as an expert witness for their candid accounts of their own loss experiences and for what I have learned from them about the richly varied realities of bereavement and the grieving that follows. Surely their stories are the heart of the matter and the point of thinking and writing about grieving at all.

In connection with my teaching I also want to thank the many colleagues with whom I have team-taught the course over the years, including Bart Gruzalski, Don Callen, Michael Allen, Donald Rothberg, Lisa Syron, Bob Strikwerda, Kathleen Dixon, Sally Fowler, and, more recently, my numerous graduate assistants for their patience and interest in what I have been attempting. Thanks are also due the administration of Bowling Green State University for supporting course development, encouraging my continued teaching and research on the subject (including providing a faculty improvement leave to enable me to finish the manuscript), and nurturing the development of an unusual department of philosophy that stresses the importance of application. Teaching about death and loss sets the teacher apart from others, yet I have never felt other than warmly embraced in my efforts. It has been a privilege.

I extend my warmest appreciation to fellow members of two

professional associations for their support and encouragement of my thinking and writing over the years. I find my professional home in the Association for Death Education and Counseling, a wonderful, warm, interdisciplinary group of dedicated professionals. Among its members I want especially to thank Terri Rando, Chuck Corr, Phyllis Silverman, Dennis Klass, Jeanne Harper, Bob Niemeyer, John Stephenson, Judy Stillion, Ben Wolfe, Hannelore Wass, Rob Stevenson, Sally Featherstone, Sandy Bertman, Larry Huston, Edie Stark, Ellen Zinner, Dick Pacholski, and Bill Worden, as well as the audiences for innumerable presentations for their encouragement over the years and for their enthusiasm for the musings of a philosopher in their midst. What a remarkable group of colleagues who are also cherished friends! I have more recently found a second professional home in the International Work Group on Death, Dying, and Bereavement. I want especially to thank Colin Murray Parkes both for his early encouragement of my professional development and for his pregnant idea that grieving involves relearning the world. I doubt that I would have written this book were it not for his influence. The idea is his, the humanities-based development here is my responsibility. Thanks are also due to my codiscussants in IWG working groups on grief and loss, including Sid and Miriam Moss, Steve Fleming, Ken Doka, Herman Monninck, and several others who have already been mentioned. What a warm, intellectually alive, and professionally responsible group.

I want to single out four professional colleagues for special recognition. First, my late teacher and friend Herbert Spiegelberg taught me the humane significance of reflection and of doing philosophy rather than simply quarreling about whether it can or must be done one way or another. I miss him. Second, Roy Nichols, funeral director and friend, has shared with my classes and workshops abundantly from his rich stock of stories of grieving persons and taught me much about the possibility and the importance of active rather than passive coping. Third, Betty Davies has been a colleague in IWG, a faithful and careful reader as the manuscript has developed, and a most enthusiastic friend and supporter throughout the writing. Indeed, she is now my wife and my life's companion. Finally, my friend and Bowling Green colleague Don Scherer has been invaluable in shaping the expression of the ideas in this book through careful reading, critical commentary, always stimulating (sometimes hysterically so) and insightful conversation, and abiding enthusiasm for carefully and caringly applying the skills of a philosopher to life in the human condition.

Despite the invention of the personal computer, we cannot function without secretaries, who deserve acknowledgement. I want to thank our Philosophy secretaries, Pat Bressler, Margy DeLuca, and Diane Petteys, for their efforts as well as for their abiding good will and patience.

Finally, I want to thank Joan Bossert, Editorial Director at Oxford, for taking a chance on a philosopher's idea and for her patience and continuing enthusiasm through the stops and starts along the way to the book's publication.

Contents

Introduction to the Revised Edition

I wanted to pack everything I could into the first edition of *How We Grieve* (1996): The best of whatever perspective and insight I had acquired from listening to stories of grieving persons all of my life. From reflection on my own loss experiences. And from teaching and writing about loss and grief for just over twenty years at that time. I thought the book might be the capstone of my writing on the subject.

The range of responses to the book has been gratifying. Leading scholars acknowledged its originality, some used it as a textbook, and many students made ample use of the ideas in the book in writing their dissertations and theses. Better yet, many counselors used the book to shape their helping efforts, some even giving copies of the book to those they serve. And, best of all, many grieving persons found it invaluable in helping them relearn the world after a loved one died.

An applied philosopher by training and aspiration, I should have known that writing the book would not put an end to my thinking about its subject. Plato once said that no one is ready to do serious philosophy until he or she is fifty. Having just crossed that milestone in 1995, I felt ready to write this book. As I look back now, I see that I was ready, and I stand by what I said then. But I also see the folly in thinking I could say something definitive. In other words, I missed the implication in Plato's remark that fifty is merely the starting point of one's best thinking. My thinking since then has continued to flow, expand, and deepen.

I was pleased when my editor at Oxford invited me to consider publishing this revised edition. I agreed with her that the text of the first edition could remain the same. We also agreed that I would concentrate my efforts on writing this new introductory essay about developments in my thinking about grieving as "relearning the world." Here I will do three things at once as I track through and comment on the six chapters of the book: I will highlight and clarify what I see as its most distinctive and still salient themes. I will elaborate on how my thinking about these themes has expanded and deepened since the first edition. And I will place my treatment of those themes in the broader context of current writings on grief and loss.

Stories of Grieving

In Chapter I, "Stories of Grieving: Listening and Responding," I begin with a brief telling of six personal stories of loss and grief, promising to tell them more fully later and to use them to ground discussions throughout the book. If any single driving force motivated me to write the book, it is an abiding conviction that personal stories are "the heart of the matter," both in responding to the bereaved and in developing thinking about grieving. I remain as passionate about this central point as I am about anything I have ever written. The existentialist philosopher in me insists that the understanding needed for a compassionate and effective caregiving response is possible only when we hear the stories grieving persons have to tell. As we listen attentively and caringly, we must focus on the uniqueness of the individual story-teller, of the challenges of living meaningfully and with integrity in his or her particular life circumstances, and of his or her personal confrontations with finiteness in bereavement and grieving.

Recently, I attended a conference presentation on grief and loss. A dear friend and colleague reported on his findings from reading a wide range of twentieth century novels by black Americans focused centrally on black characters in grief. He highlighted themes in the treatments of grieving and variations in the types of deaths, the circumstances of the deaths, and the relationships between the dead and their survivors in the novels. The stories were compelling, and discussion was very lively. Many from similar cultural backgrounds resonated with details in the stories. Others marveled at the poignancy of stories of grieving in life circumstances unfamiliar to them. Yet, some scientifically inclined members of the audience wondered about the anecdotal character of the novels and how representative they were of the experiences of grieving black populations. Others wondered about how fictional writings that do not depict real-life characters or events could serve as a basis for developing anything like a useful understanding of their subject matter.

I remember raising my hand twice to make points that I would like to repeat here. First, I urged that reading fictional (or real life) accounts of individual stories would give caregivers invaluable practice in attending carefully to the subtlety and nuance of the particularities of grieving persons' experiences. They cannot possibly do their work well if they do not become adept at doing precisely that. They do not encounter or help general populations or abstract statistics but flesh and blood individuals who live in distinctive circumstances, develop irreplaceable relationships, and have unique experiences of loss and grief. Compassionate and effective caregiving is simply not possible without the courage to engage in heart to heart dialogue with those who are suffering about what they are experiencing, listening and responding in turn. I encouraged the audience to read Rita Charon's wonderful work that stresses attunement to the singularities in personal stories and teaches valuable techniques for developing the narrative skills that caregivers need to do so.[1]

And second, I told the audience about how a Jungian analyst friend of mine had cautioned me years ago to take care in the use of the term "myth." Myths are anything but mistakes or lies, as we too often speak of them. Rather, they capture and teach us about deeply important realities of life in the human condition, sometimes grounding entire cultures in those realities. I urged the importance of getting past the idea that only scientific findings, news reports, biographies, or documentaries convey truth. Like myths, works of fiction, including folk tales, fables, parables, novels, short stories, plays, and films can be true to life without being literally true. And they can teach us a great deal about themes and narrative lines to listen for as others share their real-life tales of suffering. Full understanding requires both attunement to singularities and appreciation for the commonalities in grieving experiences.

Personal stories of loss and grief are also the heart of the matter in developing general understandings of loss and grief. Good thinking about anything requires a firm grasp on just what the thing is. The "thing itself" in the case of thinking about loss and grief is the distinctive range of human experiences that these personal stories are about. The stories are the primary means of access to those experiences. Taken together, the stories comprise the foundational evidence base in which all plausible thinking about loss and grief must take root, the data that thinking captures well or poorly. We must learn all we can about loss and grief from those who have the experiences and are able to talk about them, if we are to think in any serious way, scientific or otherwise, about the experiences.

The thinking in *How We Grieve* took root in years of listening to and reflecting on personal stories of loss and grief. Other writings in the field didn't seem to adequately reflect what I heard and observed in the experiences. I wrote the book, in part, to give abstract thinking about loss and grief a firmer foundation through description of the inherent nature of loss and grief experiences - the things themselves - the thinking should be about. *How We Grieve* offers a description and interpretation of the contours and characteristics of, or family resemblances among, experiences of loss and grief - features that make them what they are and distinguish them from other experiences. The central idea of grieving as a process of relearning the world captures not only very basic aspects of the experiences, but also their scope, complexity, multi-dimensionality, richness, and variety. And it provides general understanding of loss and grief experiences that opens the way to dialogue with grieving persons. It gives caregivers a useful framework in listening to individual stories and tuning into the particularities of personal struggles to relearn worlds of experience. The ultimate test of the validity of such descriptions and interpretations is, and always will be, whether those who experience loss and grief resonate with the general understanding they provide. The book's core descriptions and interpretations remain unchallenged in the literature. And, more significantly, caregivers and grieving persons attest that grieving involves relearning physical and social surroundings, aspects of oneself, ways of living with mystery, and ties with the deceased.

In my use of the terms bereavement, grief, and mourning are descriptions of three quite different but interrelated aspects of loss and grief. I want to be more explicit in describing what they are, since there is considerable confusion in the literature. *Bereavement* is a state of deprivation that arises after a person dies and we see his or her absence in the world of our experience as a loss. This experienced deprivation redefines and limits our life circumstances and possibilities. We relearn the world in bereavement in recognizing this life-altering change in the world as we experience it. Some write carelessly as if bereavement were a process of contending with loss when it is nothing more than the sometimes nearly unbearable recognition of it. Currently, some authors are discussing what they call "relief grief." I don't doubt that some see the absence of another as a relief, even a great relief, or that this is an experience worth taking seriously. But those who experience relief are bereaved only if they also experience deprivation. And we grieve over bereavement, not relief.

Chapter 1 affirms that we experience the impacts of bereavement as the whole persons we are. Just as we have no choice about death or bereavement, we have no choice about how they affect us. Like physical reflexes, the effects of loss come over us, though they vary far more widely from person to person than physical reflexes do. I now prefer to use the term *grief reaction* to refer to the full range of our experiences of emotional, psychological, physical, behavioral, social, cognitive, and spiritual impacts of bereavement. (In one of its uses, *mourning*, an ambiguous term, refers to what I call grief reaction.) We relearn the world in grief reactions because in them we absorb, or take in, the realities of loss for our experience of the world. I confined my use of the term *reaction* almost entirely to Chapter 2 of the book where I describe a very specific reaction that I call grief emotion. While it is a centrally important reaction to loss, it is by no means the only one. I wish I had used the term *reaction* in Chapter 5, where I talk at length about the broader range of impacts of loss as I describe the experience of the suffering that comes over us when we experience loss – including experiences of loss of wholeness and the sorrow and distress that come with it.

Many writings on grief stop short with discussions of bereavement and grief reactions, as if stories about them captured the whole of experiences of loss and grief. But, as I insist in Chapter 1 and reiterate throughout the book, grieving is not merely what happens to us as death, bereavement, and grief reactions come into our lives. Grieving is also what we do with what happens to us. Where grief reaction is passive and choiceless, the doing in grieving is active and pervaded with choice. I now prefer to use the term *grieving response* to refer to how we, again as whole persons, actively engage with bereavement and grief reaction emotionally, psychologically, cognitively, behaviorally, socially, and spiritually. We relearn the world in grieving response as through it we adapt to, and come to terms with, these changes in our worlds and the grief reactions that come over us and actively reengage in the fullness of life in a world transformed by loss. (In its second meaning, the term *mourning* also refers to what I call grieving response.) I stressed grieving response in the book to compensate for what I perceived to be both relative neglect of it in other writings or inadequate description of the nature of the labors of grieving response and their contributions to relearning the world.

I believe the most important work still to be done in developing an understanding of grief is in refining and elaborating the qualitative and descriptive thinking presented in this book. I am by no means opposed to scientific research about loss and grief when science is broadly construed to include qualitative research focused upon careful listening to personal stories of experiences after particular kinds of deaths, within specified populations, in different family or cultural contexts, in response to different caregiving efforts, and the like. Experiences of relearning, and the support offered while having them, vary a great deal, and there is so much more to be learned about these families of experience through qualitative study.

I am skeptical, however, about the statistical generalizations that issue from quantitative research in the field. To begin with, many fail to shed light on the general contours of loss and grief experiences because the instruments used measure something else entirely - for example, death anxiety or depression. Moreover, even the best of the generalizations are about probable people, not flesh and blood grieving people. The gap from generalization to application to individual cases is huge and difficult to bridge. Rarely do statistical findings provide useful insight for us individuals or our caregivers.

The most basic, traditionally scientific questions of explanation and prediction about loss and grief already have clear answers. Death of a loved one explains *bereavement* whenever it occurs. We have little problem predicting it will arise when survivors see the absence of a loved one as a loss or deprivation. The only surprises will come when we have been mistaken about who cared about or loved whom. *Grief reactions* are, in turn, explained by experiences of bereavement. We can easily predict that the bereaved will react more or less prominently in all dimensions of their being at once, as the whole persons they are. And with little more effort, we can predict that specific grief reactions will vary with the cause of death, the closeness and uniqueness of the relationship to the deceased, and the dispositions and temperaments of the bereaved.

Grieving response to bereavement and grief reaction is explained, or motivated, by those antecedent experiences. But since it is inherently active, the specific course of grieving response is unpredictable to the extent that it is shaped and colored by the individual grieving person's character and exercise of freedom and choice. We do not need quantitative research to prove that these things are true. Which is not to say that there is no need for greater understanding of them among writers and caregivers in the field. Even something as simple as the distinction between reaction and response is something that audiences find useful.

There are two areas where scientific explanation and prediction might be worth pursuing in grief research: First, it could be useful to validate or refine understanding of the causes of some of us becoming mired in grief reaction, not responding effectively or meaningfully to changes in the world of our experience and, in some instances, needing specialized professional help to relearn them. Chapter 3 implicitly identifies several such causes as it describes ways in which we are vulnerable as we grieve. In an essay written since the first edition[2] I looked at the causes of these difficulties and discussed three kinds of "extraordinary complication": (1) Aspects of our relationship with the one who died, including extreme grief emotion (discussed in Chapter 2), unfinished business with him or her, and hurtful or dysfunctional aspects of the relationship. (2) Limitations in our own abilities to relearn, including a lack of well-developed capacities to adapt and relearn the world and diagnosable psychological disorders (either pre-existing or emergent after bereavement). (3) Factors in our surrounding life circumstances, including traumatic or horrific aspects of the death, and social interactions that undermine or interfere with our grieving efforts. Perhaps research can identify other extraordinary complicating factors, or if needed, validate these ideas.

Second, it would be useful to do research to discover the causes of success or failure in approaches to caregiving, to evaluate which make things worse, which do no harm but are ineffective, and which actually help to promote effective relearning. Recently, controversy arose about whether grief counseling actually works when researchers analyzed a broad array of studies and concluded that they provide scant evidence that counseling is effective and may even do harm.[3] These latter findings were seriously challenged with argument about questionable statistical methods.[4] A deeper problem has to do with serious deficiencies in the design of the studies analyzed – small sample sizes, recruited vs. self-referred participants, heavy attrition rates, lack of controls, diffuse treatment plans and approaches examined, variations in qualifications of the counselors, lack of controls, poor outcome measure selection, etc. Clearly, research design must be refined if efforts here are to yield insights that can shape and guide effective caregiving.

Research may not yield significant results without a clear understanding of grieving as relearning the world and without means of measuring success in relearning. I am not aware of the existence of such means for carrying out this research. And without them, I strongly suspect that studies of success in grieving or caregiving are not examining the phenomena they should be examining.

Grieving Is Active

Chapter 2, "Grieving Is Active: We Need Not Be Helpless," offers a rigorous defense of the idea that grief is more than just grief reaction; it includes grieving response. That is, when we are ready to break away from whatever may be holding us in grief reaction, grieving continues as we actively engage with the realities of what has happened to us (in loss and grief reaction), and as we begin addressing challenges of relearning the world of our experience. I don't want for a minute to take back this central point about active grieving. But I do wish I had made the contrast between *reaction* and *response* more transparent and complemented the discussion of the grip of extreme grief emotion with a discussion of a broader range of grief reactions and the hold they have on us – not merely the need for ego control. I also wish I had discussed ways in which grieving response involves active engagement with grief reactions as well as reengagement with the world. And conducted the review of the history of thinking about grief in the chapter in light of these expanded discussions.

When we are bereaved, we usually grieve. But this means two fundamentally different things. On the one hand, grieving is our *reaction* when we experience the death of another as a loss. We still harbor within ourselves deeply engrained dispositions to feel, act, interact, think, expect, and hope in continuing life as if he or she were still a living presence. The powerful momentum of these dispositions still carries us into that world where we meet his or her absence nearly wherever we turn. The pain and anguish of grief reaction come over us as we realize how so many of our ways of being in the world that have become second nature to us no longer fit with the new reality where our loved one is absent. Grief reactions typically include such things as sadness, loneliness, longing, help-lessness, homesickness for the familiar, loss of courage, hope, and faith, unsettling questions and thoughts, and their somatic com-panions. These reactions happen *within* us, just as loss happens *to* us. We have no more choice about how we react to loss than we do about physical reflexes.

On the other hand, grieving is also an active *response* to both bereavement and whatever grief reaction comes over us. We engage with the death and the deprivation and changes in the world of our experience, come to terms with and even learn from our reactions to it, reshape our daily life patterns, and redirect our life stories in the light of what has happened. We respond as the multi-dimen-sional beings we are: We exert physical energy. We work through and express emotion. We change motivations, habits, and behavior patterns. We modify relationships. We return home to familiar meanings in life. We reach for inevitably new meanings. And we change ourselves in the process. Death, bereavement, and our grief *reactions* are not matters of choice. But grieving in the quite con-trasting second sense of the term as an active *response* to them is pervaded with choice. When ready, we must choose our own path in transforming the course of our lives following bereavement.

In the first edition, I went on at great length about a reaction to loss that I called "grief emotion," an emotion like no other, because at its heart is a desire for the impossible return to life of the dead. Many of us experience this emotion as the worst of grief, because within its grip we realize that the very thing we want more than any other is the one thing we cannot have. It holds a central place in grief reaction as it is nearly always felt as part of the pain that comes whenever we meet with the absence of the one we love. Spiraling down into the awful paralysis of the most extreme form of this emotion, where we doubt we can live without him or her, is one of the principal reasons why some of us become mired in grief reaction, unable to respond effectively to it without professional help. I remain convinced that this emotion stems from a desire to continue loving. But once we recognize that we can find ways of loving that do not require physical presence, we can feel the release of the grip of this emotion.

I talked about attractions of dwelling in grief emotion that can also hold us in the grip of its milder manifestations. These same attractions can hold us in the broader range of grief reactions, in-cluding holding to deeply engrained, biological attachment patterns (a kind of organic defense mechanism); hesitating in order to gather psychological strength before actively responding; resisting facing the unknown; securing secondary rewards in interactions with others; seeing intense sorrow as a way to express continuing love; and refusing to accept that life in the human condition includes limitation and vulnerability.

Since the first edition appeared, I have grown in appreciation of yet another principal way that grief reactions in general, and especially the wider range of emotions, take hold of us. I've never been happy with thinking about emotions as so many sensations or pulses of energy that pass through us with no significance in themselves. While wondering about the relation of emotion and motion, I went to the dictionary and discovered that the prefix "e" means "without" and that a root meaning of "emotion" is "without motion." Further reflection led me to realize that when emotions come over us, or tears, moans, screams, shivers, gestures, or words pour out of us, our lives stand still. Just as physical pains persist until we attend to them, emotional pains hold us motionless for good reason. We ignore or stifle emotions at our peril. More than expression, they cry out for understanding. And they persist, or grow stronger, until we pay attention to them.

When we attend to them, our emotions tell us about our brokenness, all we have taken for granted, and what we need for survival, reengaging in the world, and even thriving again. Emotions that arise from our ego tell us about our needs to be effective, desires to keep up appearances and reputation, and illusions of complete independence from others, invulnerability, and limitless control. What I choose to call emotions of soul tell us about our deep needs for roots, belonging, nurture, connection, care, and love. All of these enable us to make ourselves at home in the familiar. And what I choose to call emotions of spirit tell us about our deep needs for courage, hope, purpose, meaning, adventure, and joy. All of these enable us to reach beyond the familiar, grow, and soar in the extraordinary. When we grasp what our emotions are telling us, they loosen their grip on us and begin motivating tentative reengagement in the worlds of our experience.

About five years ago, I read Miriam Greenspan's wonderful book, *Healing Through the Dark Emotions*,[5] and was particularly taken with her idea of "befriending" what she calls "dark emotions" rather than either retreating from or trying to suppress them. Our efforts to avoid or control painful emotions are futile. She urges that there is great transformative power in emotion, if we recognize this power and allow it to work its magic within us. And she discusses several techniques that can open the way for this to happen. I don't agree that emotions work as a kind of psychological alchemy, becoming their opposites in mysterious ways when given enough time. But I have come to believe that what I call "sorrow-friendly" practices can enable us to listen effectively to our not so inscrutable emotions, learn valuable lessons from them, and use the lessons as we reengage with the world. I view these practices as grieving responses inasmuch as they provide a means of actively engaging with grief reactions. I have in mind such practices as using ceremony and ritual, sharing and exploring sorrow with another, keeping a grief journal, meditating, attending to sorrow in our bodies, pondering our dreams, calling forth and engaging with unconscious images, seeking meaning in after-death encounters with our loved ones, experiencing or creating works of art, surrendering in silence to mystery, attending to breath and breathing into deep rhythms of life, leaning into faith, and opening our hearts in prayer. For many of us, this kind of grieving response as active engagement with our grief reactions proves invaluable in readying us for active reengagement in the world.

About the same time I read Greenspan's book, I team-taught a course with the Jungian analyst I mentioned above and was taken aback when he said he was struck by how much of my book seemed focused on matters of ego. At first I resisted, but then I came to see how he could see it that way. My stressing helplessness can be taken as emphasis on ego attempts to regain control in life as soon as possible after loss. The powerlessness in extreme grief emotion, in particular, has within it a strong element of ego frustration in the face of the impossibility of returning a loved one to life. Some of the attractions of staying in our grief reaction also have aspects of ego and self-absorption in them. As written, Chapter 2 gives no clue that I see any value in lingering with, befriending, or discerning deeper needs within grief reactions. It does not discuss engaging deeper aspects of our selves, soul and spirit, as we use sorrow-friendly practices like those I mention above. And later chapters do not explicitly differentiate between ego effort and the efforts of soul and spirit involved in relearning the world.

I wish I had a vocabulary of ego, soul, and spirit available when I wrote the first edition. I would have used it to make clear a number of things: Besides ego needs, we have other, deeper needs of soul and spirit reflected in our grief reactions. Companion to ego helplessness in extreme grief emotion is a longing of soul and spirit for continuing to love in separation. The ego is also helpless in trying to deal with mysteries (suffering, death, love, and other fundamental constants in life in the human condition) as if they were problems. Our souls and spirits (mysterious themselves) are more adept at adapting to new ways of living in the human condition, pervaded with mystery as it is. Along with elements of ego that attract us to remain in grief reaction are doubts and fears of soul and spirit about their abilities to reengage in the fullness of life. Sorrow-friendly practices are both soulful (in attending to our hurt and caring about the deep needs that grief reactions reveal) and spiritual (as they support searching for meaning in grief reactions and hope and guidance for relearning the world). And soul and spirit are the principal driving forces within the self that weave and reweave the webs of our lives, move us through the unfolding of our life stories, and enable us to overcome suffering and relearn the world in the wake of bereavement – all matters discussed in later chapters.

The review of the history of thinking about grief in Chapter 2 holds up well, though, of course, there have been some developments worthy of comment here. In both thinking of grieving in terms of *stages or phases* and in *medical* terms, it is almost as if all of grieving is grief reaction – passive unfolding of experiences in predictable sequences or manifestations and then the eventual dissipation of symptoms as healing runs its course. Both ways of thinking offer only impoverished descriptions of the contours of grieving experiences and suggest that we are far more alike and predictable than we actually are. In such thinking, caregiving is limited to being present with, comforting, reassuring, and encouraging as we wait for stages or phases to pass or for treatments of symptoms to work. Neither provides entrance into dialogue about the singularities of our experiences and struggles. And some medical thinking mischaracterizes normal grief reactions as pathological.

Though most current thinking has moved past these views, there are two current developments worthy mentioning. First, the view that grieving unfolds in five stages of denial, anger, bargaining, depression, and acceptance, inadequate as it is, simply will not go away. It is nearly gospel in popular culture (among journalists, writers, and even in discussion of reactions to financial crisis!) and still too commonly used in caregiving settings. Two years ago, Elisabeth Kubler-Ross and David Kessler published a book defending the view yet again.[6] The inadequacy of the thinking is transparent when you consider how squarely focused it is on nothing other than ego flight or fight defenses and their uselessness when we contend with death and suffering. In denial, we retreat from their persistent reality.

In anger, we try to control the uncontrollable. In bargaining, we try to negotiate what cannot be changed. In depression, we concede the futility of these defenses. And when finally we reach acceptance, we grant that death and suffering are real, and implicitly acknowledge our ego's limitations. In the five-stage view, this is the end of grieving. While I will concede that many of us try to respond to death and suffering as if they were the kinds of problems or threats that egos do well with, this only adds frustration to the broader range of grief reactions we already experience. Accepting the reality of death and suffering can only be the beginning point of effective grieving response, not the end. The work of constructively engaging with our grief reactions and putting our shattered lives back together remains to be done. And our souls and spirits are far better suited for those endeavors than our egos.

Second, since the first edition appeared, many researchers have been working on defining criteria for a diagnosis of what has been variously called "pathological grief," "complicated grief," "traumatic grief," and "prolonged grief," a diagnosis intended for inclusion in the *Diagnostic and Statistical Manual* of the American Psychiatric Association. My friend and colleague, J. William Worden, does a perfectly fine job of summarizing salient features of this development and reasons for believing that some such diagnosis will be included in the next edition of the *DSM*.[7] I will only add here that I remain unconvinced that anything about grief itself is pathological. We may sometimes get into trouble and need professional help as we grieve because of extraordinary complications like those I mention above, but it is not because our grieving is a medical problem. I agree with Allan Horwitz and Jerome Wakefield[8] and with Miriam Greenspan,[9] when they argue that too much of contemporary psychology involves medicalizing even quite common human experiences such as sadness and grief. Doing so skews our understanding of the ranges of perfectly normal, though sometimes quite challenging, human experiences; stigmatizes those that have them; distorts understanding of the range of effective responses to them; and even stimulates development of drug therapies that mask them rather than confronting them. If we need help while grieving, it should be available to us without the need of a medical diagnosis. If the current system of providing care requires inappropriate diagnosis of some experiences as abnormal, there is something wrong with the system, not with those who have the experiences. Unfortunately, the system is broken in this way, and with Worden and others, I concede that getting care to those who need it takes precedence over reforming the system. Changing the *DSM*, as is being proposed, seems inevitable, and will be a bad means to this good end.

Alternatively, thinking of grieving in terms of *grief work*, rather than in terms of stages, phases, or medically, focuses on how our grieving also involves actively responding to what has happened to us. The history of thinking in this vein is on the right track in appreciating that grieving response requires active engagement with a wide range of emotional, psychological, physical, behavioral, social, cognitive, and spiritual challenges. Like all work, this engagement takes both time *and* effort. And grief work thinking is on the right track in urging that appropriate caregiving comforts us as we experience loss and absorb grief reactions, and supports us as we do the work of grieving response. I stand by what I say in Chapter 2 about these and other strengths of such thinking. And I still find great power in thinking of grieving response as relearning the world.

Respecting Individuals as They Grieve

Chapter 3, "Respecting Individuals as They Grieve," offers a deeper defense of the idea that personal stories of loss and grief are "the heart of the matter" in caregiving. Earlier I urged that no one can hope to care effectively for us as we grieve unless they attune their efforts to the singularities in what we are able to tell them about our experiences. In this chapter, I develop an ethics of care that shows how those who care for us must appreciate the details of our personal stories in order to respect us as bereaved and grieving individuals. This treatment of ethics both complements and resonates deeply with works by Arthur Frank,[10] Rita Charon,[11] and many others in the burgeoning field of narrative ethics that typically insist on the importance of attending to the particularities of our personal stories when we are ill or dying.

Chapter 3 offers ethical guidance for any who care for us as we grieve, including family members, friends, volunteers, or professionals. Those who care for us must tailor their efforts to the differences of our *needs* in bereavement, grief reaction, and grieving response. As we face the realities of loss and grief reaction, we need the understanding and compassion that can be provided by the presence of others and good listening. The presence of a caring other offers a space or context for experiencing and expressing grief reaction; assurance that our hurting matters; comfort, safety, and protection when we are vulnerable; care about our suffering; and assurance that we are embraced by community. Effective listening offers time for us to react, acceptance of our experiences, witness to our suffering, empathy and compassion, a welcoming of whatever we want to express, and interest in the stories we have to tell.

As we actively attend to and engage with our grief reactions through sorrow-friendly practices, we may need help in learning the practices themselves, guidance in our efforts, or dialogue about what we learn about our needs and possible ways of meeting them. And as we actively engage in relearning the worlds of our experience, we need help and support in meeting the distinctive challenges that physical or social surroundings, aspects of our selves, mysteries, or our relationship with the deceased present. We need help in learning to carry the pain of missing those we grieve, reshaping our daily lives, and redirecting our life stories. Such caregiving is very much like what parents, teachers, and mentors offer us when at their best in times of crisis. Those who care for us can help us to understand challenges we face, sift and choose ways of meeting them, discern hopeful possibilities for reengagement in life, continue to contend with grief reaction, reenter daily living and the next chapters of our life stories, return to the familiar, venture into the new, draw upon the best in our characters as we change ourselves and transform our lives, search for ways to love in separation, identify and adapt our responses to new faces of mystery as they present themselves, evaluate our success in relearning, learn from our mistakes, and maintain motivation when the going gets rough.

Respect for our individuality should hold a central place in caring efforts. Respect requires that those who care for us appreciate how we thrive and find meaning in life: How we have thrived in activity, experience and connection; lived with daily purpose; and found meaning in life in general, and with our loved one in particular, prior to his or her death. And how we retain the potential to thrive and live meaningfully again in the aftermath of loss. This appreciation of our past and potential thriving is not possible unless those who care for us take time to listen to the stories we have to tell. Respect also requires that those who care for us appreciate the specific ways that we are vulnerable to suffering in loss itself and vulnerable still in the circumstances within which we are grieving: How we are vulnerable to the shattering effects of loss on our daily life patterns, the disruption of the expected unfolding of our life stories, and new stresses or even breaks in our connections with things larger than ourselves. How we are vulnerable to anguish over unfinished business or even hurtful aspects of our relationship with the deceased, trauma due to the character of the death, limits in our own capacities to grieve, and disenfranchisement or other failures or dysfunctions in our relationships with fellow survivors. Once again, this appreciation of our unique vulnerabilities is not possible unless our caregivers also attend carefully to these aspects of the stories we tell them.

But respect is not merely a matter of appreciating such things about us; it also requires that those who care for us act in ways that reflect what they understand about our potential for thriving and vulnerability. Minimal respect requires that they do nothing to make things worse for us. They must do nothing to interfere in, hinder, undermine, compromise, or even block our effective response to what has happened. And authentic respect requires that those who care for us constructively support us as we engage effectively with what has happened to us in bereavement and as we struggle to relearn the world and return to thriving and living meaningfully on our own terms. Respecting our individuality, then, requires appreciation of and appropriate caring response tailored to the uniqueness of our experiences of both grief reaction and grieving response.

Correspondingly, self-respect requires that we appreciate our own potential for thriving and vulnerability, avoid making things worse for ourselves, and seek constructive means of addressing our suffering, reengaging in the world, and returning to thriving as only we can. Sorrow-friendly practices are especially powerful ways of respecting our selves as we grieve.

Disenfranchised grief[12] (the discounting or dismissal of grief) is a topic I have explored further since the first edition appeared.[13] Invoking the ethic of respect for individuality in grieving, I argued that disenfranchisement is not merely a failure of empathy as professional colleagues have suggested,[14] a view that captures only failure to appreciate our vulnerability and suffering. Instead, I urge that it is profoundly disrespectful in making things worse for us. Disenfranchisement is actively destructive as messages discount, dismiss, disapprove, discourage, invalidate, and delegitimate our experiences. And as behaviors interfere with the exercise of our right to grieve by withholding permission, disallowing, constraining, hindering, and even prohibiting it. The deep ethical offense in disenfranchising lies in how it withholds support from, breaks connections with, isolates, and abandons us when we are hurting.

In that article, I also note that virtually all writings on the subject focus on disenfranchising bereavement and grief reaction, a limitation I attribute to lack of widespread understanding of the distinction between reaction and response in writings on loss and grief. I urge that the scope of disenfranchisement extends to grieving response as well. Messages and behaviors also disenfranchise our striving to transcend suffering and return to thriving. I focus on how, in particular, they disenfranchise hope (a core aspect of our resilience) and love in separation (a central feature of relearning the world). And I elaborate on constructive ways of respectfully supporting hope and love.

I have also elaborated my thinking on respect for grieving individuals in three other papers: One[15] is about respect for bereaved children and adolescents, highlighting their distinctive ways of thriving and finding meaning in their experiences, their unique vulnerabilities, and respectful ways of helping them contend with suffering and relearning their worlds. The second[16] describes the existential suffering of children, our strong tendencies to discount even the possibility that they are susceptible to such suffering, and respectful ways of helping them in the throes of such suffering. And the third[17] explores what respect for the spiritual beliefs of the dying and bereaved requires.

Relearning the World

Chapter 4, "Relearning the World," fleshes out a distinctive account of grieving response as nothing less than relearning the world of our experience. Our relearning may or may not involve using sorrow-friendly practices to learn from our bereavement and grief reactions. Some of us do better than others in sensing what we need to do in order to reengage in the world and, when we are ready, doing it straightforwardly without self-consciously pausing or reflecting.

One of the most stunning misinterpretations of grieving as relearning the world mistakes it as cognitive, or at least primarily so. From the very beginning, I discuss the difference between (1) thinking of relearning as *learning that* a loved one has died, and *that* the world is different in many ways because of it, and (2) thinking of relearning as *learning how* to be and act in a world where that event and those changes have come into our lives. I describe in great detail how relearning the world is a multi-dimensional process of learning *how* to live meaningfully again after loss. To be sure, this relearning is partly cognitive, but that is by no means the whole, nor the most important part, of it. But still, too many readers drift toward that troubling misinterpretation.

Let me tell a story that makes the difference between learning *that* and learning *how* transparent. In the nineteenth century, when bicycles came into fashion, an amazing thing happened. Authors began writing and selling huge numbers of books *about* how to ride the new contraptions, some even exceeding five hundred pages. There were reading groups and classes centered on the books and learning from them *that* riding a bicycle requires mounting, achieving and maintaining balance, steering, respecting momentum, braking, dismounting without falling, and so forth. You can imagine, I am sure, that novices knew nothing more whatever about *how* to ride a bicycle after reading any or all of the books. And you can picture, I am also sure, what happened when they first tried to ride.

Although many of us benefit from reading books about others' personal experiences of loss or ways of thinking about the experiences, we do eventually have to find the courage, faith, and hope we need to reengage in the world, take tentative first steps, try, fail, try again, fail better, and eventually relearn *how* to be and act in the world that loss changed so profoundly. Relearning the world after a loved one dies is learning *how* to live in balance again, not learning *that* you will have to do so.

When I first began thinking and teaching about loss and grief thirty-five years ago, the focus in writing and caregiving fell on the affective dimension of our experiences. Emotions were not understood as reflections of our deep needs, but they were the heart of what grieving was thought to be. And being present with and comforting those in their thrall and as they dissipated over time was the be all and end all of caregiving. There was some thinking about our active engagement with loss (grieving response), but it was overwhelmed by the emphasis on affect and grief reaction. There was little, if any, appreciation of the power of the mind to adapt to new realities. Some of my early teaching aimed at underscoring how valuable the mind is in helping us to understand and orient ourselves in reality, especially when loss changes it so profoundly. The power of reflection is surely one of the things that make sorrow-friendly practices, including counseling with another, effective.

Over time, the pendulum may have swung too far in the other direction, as cognition now seems too heavily emphasized. It is heartening to see fuller appreciation of the cognitive dimension of grieving in a new emphasis on meaning-making and narrative therapy. But while the labors of grieving through relearning the world have a cognitive dimension, shifting our thinking, even revising the stories that we tell ourselves about our lives and the world around us, it is not the heart of grieving. Insights gained from telling our stories, attending to our grief reactions, and reflecting can, at their best, provide guidance in doing the multi-dimensional work of re-learning the world.

To better understand grieving response as relearning (or reen-gagement with) the world, it is helpful to consider how we learn our way in (engage with) the world in the first place. I follow philoso-pher Martin Heidegger[18] in thinking of human existence as caring engagement in the world around us, a world best thought of as the field of our experiences. His reading of "caring engagement" em-phasizes our pragmatic involvement in life projects, meeting practi-cal problems and challenges, and overcoming obstacles. I read "care" more broadly to include what I call our soulful engagement in receiving from and giving to others in respect, love, friendship, and compassion and in making ourselves at home in our surround-ings. I also read "care" to include what I call our spiritual engage-ment in venturing into the new, reaching for the extraordinary, seeking growth, searching for transcendent understanding of how to live meaningfully, and striving to live meaningfully, sometimes through spiritual practice. We are primarily caring beings intention-ally alive within our surroundings, and usually, but not always, ca-pable of self-awareness and reflection when necessary. *Learning how* to practically, soulfully, and spiritually engage situates and ori-ents us in the world of our experience at the deepest level and shapes our lives.

From our earliest moments, before we have language or capaci-ties to reflect or deliberate, we experience the world as sometimes nourishing, sometimes barren; sometimes comforting, sometimes hostile; sometimes interesting, sometimes not so interesting; some-times supportive, sometimes challenging; sometimes open, some-times closed. Over time we learn how to be and act in the world, as we satisfy our pragmatic, soulful, and spiritual needs and desires; broaden our experiences; become involved in activities; pursue in-terests; find places for ourselves in our physical surroundings; walk the earth beneath the sun and stars; connect in relationships with others, families, and communities; and engage with mystery. We involve ourselves straightforwardly in the richness and diversity of the world. We weave unique daily life patterns. And we live out and embody unique life stories. Through caring engagement we "as-sume" places in the world; we become caught up in living in it.

We establish and orient ourselves in the world in and through the needs, wants, emotions, motivations, abilities, habits, dispositions, interaction patterns, expectations, and hopes that arise within and shape our caring engagement with it. Only rarely do we reflect, theorize, or self-consciously plan and strategize. *Learning that,* in other words, comes after and is often reflexively about *how* to be and act in the world. *Learning that* is most commonly motivated when straight-ahead engagement in the world doesn't suffice in meeting our needs, fulfilling our desires, meeting challenges, or the like. *Learning that* is validated by, and grounded in, the full range of experiences of caring engagement in the world. It aims importantly at understanding the fields of our experience and our selves in those experiences. And it sometimes serves as a foundation for more deliberate planning of changes in our life course.

Loss of the assumptive world that comes with bereavement is an area I have explored more fully since the first edition appeared.[19] I argue that the assumptions undone by bereavement are not only, or even primarily, cognitive assumptions. Commonly, when we assume, we take something for granted without really thinking about it at all. The cognitive view of assumptions misses the *learning how* to live in the world that takes place at a fundamentally deeper level in our lives, beneath the gaze of our reflective awareness, prior to self-conscious thought and deliberation. Bereavement catches us up short, leaving us poised to continue in ways we have known *how* to live in a changed world where, in so many ways, we now don't know at all *how* to live. Bereavement renders useless all we have learned about *how* to live in the presence of our loved one. And it unsettles our confidence in what we have learned about *how to live* with everything that reminds us of our separation from him or her in our physical and social surroundings and within ourselves. Many of us are not at all sure about *how*, or even whether, we can live meaningfully without our loved one's precious presence. Bereavement undermines our ego's practical functioning and self-confidence: We are not sure of *how* to carry on with the details and problems of daily life, especially the unexpected and unwelcome changes in them. Bereavement uproots our souls: We don't know quite *how* to trust what remains of the familiar, make ourselves at home again in the world, or live with and love others who survive with us. And bereavement shakes our spirits: We don't know just *how* to find meaning in living again, enter unanticipated chapters of our life stories, or find the courage, hope, and faith we need to stretch into an inevitably new world. To be sure, in lifetimes of learning *how to live* in the world, we also come to believe *that* the world is more or less safe and just, and *that* our place in it is more or less secure. Bereavement also causes many of us to doubt what we had taken for granted in these understandings of the nature of the world itself. For most of us, this unsettling of our beliefs, painful as it can be, is only part, and not the most important part, of the loss of assumptive world we experience in bereavement. The visceral unsettling of the sense that there is a place where we belong in the great scheme of things is far worse. The labors of grieving include relearning all of what bereavement unsettles about what we have taken for granted about *how to live.*

Relearning the world is not merely, or even centrally, addressing and solving problems. We usually reengage in living about as reflectively and deliberately as we engaged in living in the first place. Only occasionally, when we sense we are up against something we need to think about, do we switch into problem-solving mode where we self-consciously sort through alternative perspectives to address the challenges before us. "Problem-solving" also suggests that grieving is a matter of *addressing tasks* - bits of work that can be completed. Relearning aspects of our physical surroundings, social surroundings, and selves often has this character as we make rather small-scale (though by no means easy) adjustments in living. For example, we see a father's favorite chair in a new light, approach a fellow survivor with a memory to share, or let go of a habit that requires the physical presence of the one who died.

But over time, as we address many tasks in the particular corners of our worlds, we also cumulatively accomplish other things: We take in the reality of loss (modify our understanding). We experience, express, and are guided by emotion that bereavement arouses (adjust emotionally). We change how we inhabit surroundings that echo with loss (modify behavior and relationships). And we find ways of loving in separation from our loved one (modify that singular relationship). Neither problem-solving nor completing tasks, these aspects of grief work are far better understood as dimensions of human life and grieving. Typically, we do them together rather than in isolation from one another; we grieve as whole persons. For example, in the case of a father's chair, relearning is all at once a matter of realizing that he will never sit in it again; feeling, expressing, and being guided by a range of emotions; deciding how to behave around the chair or what to do with it; negotiating with other family members who may have other preferences about the chair; and experiencing connection with father in a new way. And coming to terms with loss in any of these dimensions is clearly more like engaging in *life-long projects* than completing a circumscribable bit of work. We never finish life-long projects of taking in the realities of loss, accommodating emotionally to them, changing our behaviors and reshaping our lives, or adapting our relationship with our loved one as we do with true "tasks."[20]

As we grieve, we also engage with some of the most profound mysteries of life, including finiteness and limitation, change and impermanence, uncertainty, fallibility, vulnerability and suffering, death and mortality, the depths of soul and spirit (our own and others'), love and relationship, and the meaning of life. *Engaging with mystery* is neither problem-solving nor completing tasks. None of these mysteries can be solved, answered definitively, controlled, managed, or mastered. We never finish with any of them or deal with them decisively. They are constants in our surroundings, conditions of ongoing living that persistently challenge and provoke us, especially when we are bereaved. They present themselves in ever-changing perspectives that reveal often new, provocative facets of life that transcend our understanding. We cannot change them (though our egos may try). We can only change in response to them. Some responses are more sustainable than others, some more suited to some of us than others. Our responses are always provisional, subject to change. Our souls and spirits dance with them as long as we live.

Grieving as meaning-making is another topic I have explored since the first edition appeared.[21] The term "making" here suggests that we are self-consciously active, take deliberate initiative, and bring new meanings into existence as we grieve. I agree that, as we grieve, we sometimes give meaning to our experiences and actions, and especially to our suffering; often read new meanings into or off of our surroundings; self-consciously reshape patterns of meaning in our daily lives; deliberately plan and venture forth on new, and hopefully meaningful, life courses; restructure and reinterpret aspects of our life narratives and the self-understandings based in them; and reevaluate, and often modify, our understandings of our place in the larger scheme of things.

But, this view of grieving misses how much of what we do as we grieve is a matter of meaning-finding. "Finding" here suggests that at other times we are less self-conscious in what we do, are more passive or receptive, and return to or encounter something already established, and often not of our own doing, as we mourn. We unreflectively return to experiences and actions that hold familiar meanings. We become aware of and accept meanings that seem to arise spontaneously in our suffering. We find our way home within surroundings filled with well-established meanings. We find we can trust elements of our daily life patterns that remain viable. We find that some long-held hopes and aspirations still move us down familiar life paths. We recognize meaningful continuity in our life narratives and the characters we embody in them. And we often deepen our appreciation of familiar understandings of our place in the larger scheme of things.

In recent years, much attention has been paid to a "dual-process model" of grieving[22] that focuses on the stressors in grieving response. The model distinguishes between "loss-oriented" stressors and "restoration-oriented" stressors. Loss-oriented stressors have to do with our loved one and dealing with the pain of separation, realizing what loss means to us, and finding a new place for him or her in a world where he or she is no longer present. Restoration-oriented stressors, supposedly by contrast, have to do with mastering skills, changing our identities, making a variety of psychological and social transitions in living, and modifying our thinking about our selves and reality. The proponents of the dual-process model say it is not possible to attend to both kinds of stressor at once and that we must deal with both to respond effectively to loss. The key idea is that we will do best when we *oscillate* between these two kinds of stressors, engaging with one and avoiding the other, and, over time, going back and forth.

I could understand if the view was a suggestion to go back and forth between engagement with grief reaction, perhaps through sorrow-friendly practices, and grieving response where we use what we learn from grief reaction. We would learn a bit, then give it a try; if it works, go back to learn something else; if it doesn't work, go back and probe more deeply; and the like. But proponents seem to have in mind stressors that arise not as we engage with grief reaction but rather as we actively engage with different aspects of the wider world. Where loss stressors center on relearning our relationship with the deceased, restoration stressors center on relearning the rest of our world, including our selves.

But, in most experiences of grieving response, we address the pain of separation and other aspects of our ties with our loved one precisely in experiences of engaging with the aspects of the world that remind us of him or her - that is, nearly everywhere. Think of the father's chair in the earlier example. The mourner meets with both loss and restoration stressors at once in that experience. Whether, or how, to rearrange the furniture or whether and when to sit in the chair are (restoration) issues only *because* the chair belonged to the father and it simultaneously reminds his survivors of separation from him (loss). More often than not, the stressful aspects of relearning the world arouse loss-oriented and restoration-oriented stress simultaneously, not in isolation from one another. So the oscillation recommendation seems to have, at best, limited application.

Relearning Our Selves

In Chapter 5, "Relearning Our Selves: Grief and Personal Integrity," I offer a unique discussion of loss and grief that delves into the nature of our selves and our suffering and the effects of suffering on our identity and personal integrity. If our selves were self-contained social atoms, isolated in their development, impermeable and invulnerable, and truly independent, as so many commonly think, we would not be shattered by the loss of someone we care about or love. His or her death would simply be a matter of the disappearance of another nearby self-contained being. We would remain entirely intact. But the truth of the matter is that loss shakes our personal integrity and identity. Bereavement penetrates to the core of our being.

I develop a different metaphor for the nature of the self that accounts for these shattering effects of bereavement. It is better to think of our self as a web of caring engagements with, and connections to, elements in the world around us. This self, in turn, is enmeshed within a web of webs encompassing our families and communities, the surrounding world, and ultimately all that is. We all know how much our relationships matter to us, "everything" to some. But few of us ever stop to think of how the connection and grounding that such relationships afford are integral to our being who we are. In our unique personal histories of weaving and reweaving patterns of caring connection within intimate and broader social contexts and in the wider world, our self-images, self-concepts, self-confidence, self-esteem, personal integrity, and personal identity emerge. We are the individuals we are by virtue of the distinctive life patterns, or webs of life, we establish as we caringly engage in the world. Our selves are by their nature social, permeable, and interdependent. This makes us vulnerable to the loss of wholeness and to the pain and anguish which bereavement entails. Loss pierces our hearts *because* we were intimately connected to our loved one in innumerable ties; *because* we were anything but separate.

When a loved one dies, it feels as if we are falling apart. Bereavement is like a shattering blow to the web of our caring engagements in the world, to our very selves as we experience them. The worst of our brokenness is the awful and pervasive sense of separation from our loved one. Our illusions of independence, control, and invulnerability are shattered. And we experience brokenness in our daily life patterns, life stories, and connections with larger wholes. Loss unravels our daily life pattern: It can never be just as it was before the death. The extent of the devastation in the web is proportionate to the prominence of the place in daily life held by our loved one. Many of the feelings, desires, motivations, dispositions, habits, and expectations that shaped daily life when he or she lived remain within us but no longer cohere with reality. Loss disrupts our life story, again more or less profoundly, depending on how central a place our loved one held in it. The next chapters cannot unfold just as we expected, hoped, or dreamed they would. Its coherence and meaning are threatened. And loss threatens or undermines the wholeness that derives from our being part of larger wholes. Ties with family and community are strained. We can feel out of place within them and no longer at home in the greater scheme of things.

Our suffering has a terrible inertia. When we find ourselves in the midst of brokenness, pain, and anguish after loss, we experience ourselves as victims, passive recipients of unwelcome impositions in our lives. We feel helpless, powerless before forces larger than ourselves. We become preoccupied and humbled by events and consequences beyond our control, frightened by our own seeming smallness and insignificance. We sense that our losses are irretrievable, that we can no longer find meaning, realize value, or know love now that the one we love is dead and cannot return to us. We fear that our distress is without end and that our agony is constant and unrelenting. We fear that life on the far side of our present, pervasive agony is unimaginable and that meaning, joy, and love will forever elude us. We lose motivation and are at a loss as to what to do or say that can make any difference. We desperately need to move in a positive direction through and beyond the worst of our agony, but we are at a loss as to what that direction might be.

As we grieve in response to our brokenness, we reweave the web of our caring engagements in the world, and, in the process, relearn ways of being our selves. Our reweaving changes the patterns of the threads of our caring connections to things, places, experiences, activities, other individuals, family, and community, and our sense of place in the greater scheme of things. Our reweaving also takes our life story in new directions, changing its plot, subplots, and themes as well as roles that our fellow survivors, newcomers, and we play. As we reweave with others, changing patterns of caring connection among us and our family and community histories, we learn new ways of being with one another. Our web's new pattern and unfolding story support a new identity, embody a new integrity, and reflect changes in our character. Our reweaving, when it goes well, carries us past the inertia of our suffering, heals our brokenness, and revives the flow of life along the lifelines that comprise the web.

I find the web metaphor provides a powerful and accessible perspective on the emergence of our sense of self, bereavement, grief reaction, and grieving response. Yet, from the time when I first drew atoms and webs on the blackboard while teaching, I was at a loss for vocabulary to describe the forces deep within our self that do the weaving and reweaving. Only while writing my second book,[23] did the words come to me. I now use the term "soul" to refer to the "home-seeking" aspect of our self that is the driving force within us - an aspect of our will to live - that seeks nurture, connection, and grounding in the familiar. Where it finds these things, it offers care, love, and compassion in return. And I use the term "spirit" to refer to the "meaning-seeking" aspect of our self. It is the driving force within us - another aspect of our will to live - that reaches for the new and extraordinary in adventure, growth, and joy, strives to overcome adversity, and searches for transcendent understanding. Our soul anchors the web of our life within the larger network of webs that makes up our world. And our spirit reweaves the web in response to change, opportunity, and challenge. Our soul's cares and loves and our spirit's faith, hope, and courage make us who we are. Together, soul and spirit comprise the depth of our character.

Most of the time, as I said above, the weaving and reweaving of the web of caring engagements in the world by soul and spirit is accomplished straightforwardly and not self-consciously. Only in unusual circumstances, commonly when things aren't going well or we are in crisis, do we become aware of the usually anonymous operations of soul and spirit in our lives and reflect on their needs and how to meet them. Our ego, however, is quite different. In many ways, it is usually self-conscious as it goes after what it wants; solves everyday practical problems; competes for attention and advantage; concerns itself with appearance, success, and reputation; develops illusions of control and complete independence from others; and defends against perceived threats to control and separateness, sometimes even stifling awareness of the powerful forces of soul and spirit within us. Our ego functions on the surface of the web of our life while blissfully unaware of the ongoing anonymous functioning of soul and spirit in weaving and reweaving the web on which it depends.

In bereavement, we are suspended between a life we knew with our loved one and the daunting unknown of life in separation from him or her. Profound change in the world calls for profound change in us. But our ego, soul, and spirit are all in crisis. Our disillusioned ego is helpless before events it could not, and mysteries it cannot, control. Our soul is uprooted and wrenched out of the familiar, doubting if it can ever care so deeply or feel at home again. And our spirit is fearful and discouraged, doubting if it can overcome sorrow, face unwelcome change, or ever know meaning, love, or joy again.

In relearning the world, we relearn these aspects of our self. We relearn the ways of our ego as we begin again to solve everyday problems, control what is ours to control, and navigate effectively in practical ways. Greater awareness of the depth of our being and interdependence, if we come to it, enables us to resist our ego's tendencies to illusion and control. We relearn the ways of our soul as we begin again to draw support from roots and connections already in place, pour our love and care into the familiar, and make ourselves at home again in our daily life. And we relearn the ways of our spirit as we begin to reweave the web of our daily life, joining new threads of caring engagement with the familiar; reach past our hurt and enter the unknown with courage, faith, and hope; and find and make fresh meanings in the next chapters of our life story.

Through loss and suffering, we may even develop new strength of character, as we grow in self-understanding and appreciation of our soul and spirit. As we become more sensitive and responsive to others. As we learn how much others mean to us, and new ways to show gratitude and love. Or as we gain critical perspective on reality and life in the human condition.

Writers and researchers have turned their attention recently to resilience in grieving,[24] attending to the majority of us who grieve relatively successfully and, usually, neither need nor reach out for help. What is it about these more resilient among us that makes them so? I want to suggest here that our resilience resides in what is not broken. To be sure, our daily lives are shattered, our life stories disrupted, our connections to larger wholes threatened or undermined, and our ego's illusions undone. Yet, much in the tattered web of our life remains intact. Much good in the web of webs that has supported us throughout our lives remains available. And neither our soul nor spirit is broken. The home-seeking and meaning-seeking drives that animate our lives, though shaken, can and do address our brokenness and overcome our sorrow. Resilient souls find sustenance in familiar surroundings; draw from roots in family, community, history, and tradition; care and love deeply; and find grounding in the great scheme of things. Resilient spirits find hope, faith, and courage to rise above suffering; stretch into the new and unknown; change and grow; seek understanding; and open to joy again. And the love that still pulses in our soul and spirit can cherish precious memories and lasting legacies, revive connections with fellow survivors, and open to new relationships. As our unbroken and resilient soul and spirit do these things we relearn how to be our selves again in life in separation from our loved one.

Relearning Our Ties with the Deceased

Chapter 6, "Relearning Our Ties with the Deceased: Grief, Love, and Separation," urges that labors of love are at the heart of our relearning the world. Nothing is more important, difficult, or potentially rewarding for us than learning how to continue loving in separation. The chapter describes how we can continue loving and how doing so is good for both those we mourn and us.

When a loved one dies, we want still to experience the warmth of his or her care and love for us and to continue caring about and loving him or her. If bereavement is about our loss and grief reaction about our missing the one we mourn, then grieving response is about our hope. We labor in grieving in order to rise above our suffering and reaffirm meaning in life. Hope is the will to do so. In hope we open and make ourselves ready to welcome unexpected possibilities and pursue meaning down unanticipated pathways. Searching for lasting love in separation is our best hope for transcending suffering and reaffirming the continuing meanings of the life now ended and of our own. I felt these matters were so important that I devoted my entire second book[25] to the themes introduced in this chapter, showing, largely through stories, how we can find hopeful paths and how caregivers can support our labors of love.

We should never underestimate the importance of what we have lost. The presence of, and sharing life with, those we love is precious. We learn this when in bereavement and grief reaction we realize how much we have taken for granted and when in relearning the world we meet their absence nearly everywhere we turn. Yet, paradoxically, we gain a vital perspective on our suffering when we remember that we should not overestimate what we have lost. The lives of those we have loved were, and remain, real for us. We retain our unique acquaintance with them. Their deaths do not cancel the days they walked with us. The times we spent together with them are not erased from history. We still hold memories that we can share with fellow survivors and others. And we still hold much of what those we have loved have given. We still feel the imprint of their lives upon our practical lives and our characters, in our souls and spirits. We still hold the legacies of their lives, the differences they made in our individual, family, and community lives while here. When we realize these things, we begin to sense how we may "let go" of what we have lost (their presence) and begin to move toward cherishing what we still have of them. We retain our capacities to sense abiding love from, and to love in return, those who have died. We experience their continuing love for us as we realize all they have given and continue to give. And we express our love for them as we cherish their memories and embrace life lessons they have taught us.

This thinking counters longstanding theory and counseling practice that promoted complete detachment or "letting go" of emotional ties to the deceased. It is a shame that theory and practice went as far astray as they did. That they had done so was confirmed when, in the same year *How We Grieve* appeared, colleagues of mine published what was then received, and is still now thought of, as a groundbreaking work about what they called "continuing bonds" with those who die.[26] I was amazed when they wrote that "research results were beginning to reveal" that such continuing bonds exist. I couldn't help wondering if they had ever listened to stories of loss and grief told by the bereaved like those I've heard all my life and that counselors hear every day, stories that almost invariably explore memories of the deceased. Or whether there was never any remembering of, or talk about the dead, in their homes or families. Or if they were so distant from traditions that they missed how traditional beliefs and practices support lasting love of founding figures and connection with, and even reverence for, ancestors. Or whether the psychiatrists among them had never dealt with clients struggling with issues with long-dead parents. The continuing disconnect between some research in the field and the stories of lasting love told by so many became transparent to me shortly after

I published *The Heart of Grief* four years later. I had sent a copy to a prominent psychiatrist friend. When next we met, he told me with great enthusiasm that the stories in it captured "everything we see in our counseling practice," but added only a moment later, "Now all we need is the research to prove that it is true."

Insistence on complete emotional detachment appears to have been motivated by belief or fear that continuing ties to the deceased can only be morbid. But it is a mistake to think that anything associated with death is by definition morbid. Rather, something is morbid only if it compromises our thriving; drains our life of its value, purpose and meaning; or perpetuates our suffering. Let's look at the possibilities for morbidity in attachment to those we mourn: It is clear that the desire for an impossible return of our loved one can become morbid when our simple and harmless wishing for it becomes fervent and preoccupying desire. But the desire for lasting love implicit in our desire for a return is not morbid. It can motivate us to do things that lead to its fulfillment. Fulfilling it enhances and enriches our lives as we retrieve precious memories and embrace valuable legacies. And it leads us to hope, not despair.

We know much about non-morbid love in separation. Love in separation is essential in virtually all of our loving relationships when both parties are alive. We spend a great deal, or even most, of our time apart from those we love. And there is much positive, life-enhancing, meaningful give and take without physical presence. We do not stop loving or being loved when we part. For example, we remember and speak of, take delight in, cry with, express affection for, voice concern for, do things for, keep promises to, feel comforted or encouraged by, draw inspiration from, try to be more like, praise and feel grateful for one another when we are apart.

We also know much about what is good or troubling in our loving and caring ties with others. Though morbidity, or trouble, is often part of ties among the living, it does not follow that all such ties are morbid. And we know a great deal about avoiding or overcoming trouble in ties with the living. Just as morbidity is avoidable in those ties, so it is avoidable in ties to the deceased.

In first encounters with our physical surroundings, social surroundings, and aspects of our selves, we are reminded painfully of the absence of our loved one almost everywhere we turn. Though we are inclined to retreat from painful reminders, they are inescapable. We are reminded of our loved one's absence precisely *because* so much in the world of our experience has been touched and imbued with meaning by the life and character of the one we mourn.

Paradoxically, the very same elements in living that remind us of absence also hold precious memories and legacies. By no means easy at first, we can reach past the pain of separation and affirm the abiding meanings and continuing presence of our loved one in memory and legacy. We can then cherish their memories and embrace their legacies, using valuable lessons in living or constructively identifying with some of their cares, interests, or traits of soul and spirit. Much of learning to carry the residual pain of missing our loved one involves becoming more adept at allowing the pain of separation to recede to the background and keeping positive memory and appreciation of legacy in the foreground of our experience.

Reaching through pain in this way is clearly illustrated in a recent video I viewed of a therapy session with a woman whose young son had died.[27] The therapist had asked her to bring in something her son had given her. When she shows him her son's gift, she weeps, missing him terribly. Kindly acknowledging her pain, the therapist asks her gently about the circumstances when her son gave her the object. As she tells the story, she remembers details of a good time in their lives together, delights in them again, and says how much she always appreciated her son's thoughtfulness and generosity. As she grows animated in the telling, her tears vanish. By the time she finishes, she is actually laughing with her therapist. And it is no stretch at all to say that she enjoys her son again, laughing with him, too.

Lasting love is not only possible, but it is desirable both for our loved ones and for us. Lasting love is good for our loved ones as it furthers some of their interests and fulfills their desire to make lasting differences while they are here. It also fulfills their desires that we live well and hold dear the good in their lives. And it gives them a kind of symbolic immortality, an abiding meaning not touched by death. Lasting love is also good for us who mourn them, as remembering the good in life with them and embracing their legacies enriches our lives. It fulfills our desire to still love them without falling into the futility of desiring their return, giving them a different kind of presence in our lives. It helps us to find meaning in our suffering, making us whole again as we weave their legacies into our daily lives, carry them with us into the next chapters of our life stories, and hold them dear as part of our families and communities. Cherishing their legacies mitigates the pain of missing them, making it more like the pain of separation when they were alive.

Since the first edition appeared, I published an essay about anticipatory grief and starting the transition to loving in separation while our loved ones are dying.[28] Much early writing insisted that anticipatory grief is harmful because it involves premature "letting go", even abandonment, of the dying. But, when properly understood, anticipatory grief has nothing to do with such detachment. Rather, anticipatory grief is the grieving that we do together with our loved ones while we anticipate their dying and our life after their death. We grieve together over losses already experienced during the dying process and anticipate loss and sorrow to come. We do what we can to finish unfinished business and live out as well as possible our last days together. And we take the first steps in a transition from loving in presence to loving in separation, anticipating how to balance the pain to come of missing our loved one with cherishing their memories and legacies.

Remembering with the dying provides opportunities to express our love for one another and gratitude for our life together and all it has given us. Anticipating the future together allows us to discuss ways in which we can further their desires and interests in what matters most to them after they die. We can make promises to them and assure them that we will abide by long-standing covenants between us. We can tell them how we will cherish them in memory. We can let them know how we are different and enriched for having known them. We can tell them how we will use and cherish the legacies of their practical influence, what they have taught us about living with care and love, and the inspiration that they have given us. We can pledge to strive to realize the hopes they have for us as individuals, families, and communities. And we can assure them that we will do our best to balance the pain of missing them with loving them in separation in all of these ways.

In Closing

It seems fitting to draw this essay to a close with a brief discussion of closure. It is no more plausible to think that grieving ends in closure than that it ends in a "fifth stage" of acceptance, the recognition that loss is real. Yet, the idea persists in popular culture and everyday understanding. At its worst, the idea of closure gives rise to unrealistic expectations in us and our caregivers about what is possible, expectations bound to be disappointed. Striving for closure diverts attention from the real challenges in relearning the world.

Of course, we do bring to a close some of what we experience and do while we grieve. For example, we spend time with our loved one's body; notify others about what has happened; make it through rituals and ceremonies; file legal papers and settle estates; decide what to do with things left behind; go into rooms or to places we have avoided; accept kind gestures from others; write thank-you notes; have difficult conversations; find answers to concrete questions about what happened or who, if anyone, was responsible; return to work or activities that still matter to us; or finish some unfinished business with our loved one. In these experiences and efforts, and so many others like them, we find small measures of closure as we complete tasks, address problems, and make decisions. But none bring our grieving to a close.

When you think of the scale of it, it makes no more sense to think that we complete relearning the world after loss than that we complete learning the world period. It is, after all, a world that we learn and relearn. And the learning and relearning both involve learning *how to live*. Few of us ever think we are done learning how to live. And if we do think we are, something always comes along to show us how foolish we are. When you think about specific labors of relearning, it becomes even more obvious that closure will always elude us. We never finish with life-long projects of taking in the realities of the world and of loss, accommodating emotionally to them, changing our behaviors and reshaping our life patterns, or adapting our relationship with our loved one, before or after he or she dies. Though his or her life ends at death, our relationship does not. We will never stop missing our loved one, but instead learn to carry the pain. And we will never stop loving him or her, but instead learn how to continue loving in separation. The dances of our souls and spirits (the mysteries within us) with surrounding mystery never end as we meet new faces and challenges that limitation, change, fallibility, uncertainty, suffering, death, love, and the souls and spirits of those we love and mourn present. We don't change these realities but instead continue living, changing, and grieving in response to them as long as we live.

Notes

1. Rita Charon, *Narrative Medicine: Honoring the Stories of Illness* (New York: Oxford University Press, 2006).

2. Thomas Attig, "Relearning the World: Always Complicated, Sometimes More Than Others," in *Complicated Grieving and Bereavement: Understanding and Treating People Experiencing Loss*, ed. G. R. Cox, R. A. Bendiksen, and R. G. Stevenson (Amityville, New York, Baywood Publishing, 2001): 7–19.

3. John Jordan and Robert Neimeyer, "Does Grief Counseling Work? *Death Studies, 27* (2003): 765–786.

4. Dale Larson and W. Hoyt, "What has become of grief counseling: An evaluation of the empirical foundations of the new pessimism. *Professional Psychology,: Research and Practice, 38* (2007): 347–355.

5. Miriam Greenspan, *Healing through the Dark Emotions: The Wisdom of Grief, Fear, and Despair* (Boston, Massachusetts: Shambhala Publications, 2003).

6. Elisabeth Kubler-Ross and David Kessler, *On Grief and Grieving: Finding the Meaning of Grief through the Five Stages of Loss* (New York: Scribner's, 2007).

7. J. William Worden, *Grief Counseling and Grief Therapy, Fourth Edition* (New York: Springer Publishing Company, 2009): 135–137.

8. Alan V. Horwitz and Jerome C. Wakefield, *The Loss of Sadness: How Psychiatry Transformed Normal Sorrow into Depressive Disorder* (New York: Oxford University Press, 2007).

9. Miriam Greenspan, *Healing through the Dark Emotions.*

10. Arthur Frank, *At the Will of the Body: Reflections on Illness* (Boston: Houghton-Mifflin, 1991), *The Wounded Storyteller: Body, Illness, and Ethics* (Chicago: University of Chicago Press, 1995), and *The Renewal of Generosity: Illness, Medicine, and How to Live* (Chicago: University of Chicago Press, 2004).

11. Rita Charon, *Narrative Medicine,* Chapter 10: "The Bioethics of Narrative Medicine," 203–218.

12. Kenneth Doka, ed., *Disenfranchised Grief: New Directions, Challenges, and Strategies for Practice* (Champaign, Illinois: Research Press, 2002).

13. Thomas Attig, "Disenfranchised Grief Revisited: Discounting Hope and Love," *Omega* xx (2004): 197–215.

14. Robert Neimeyer and John Jordan, "Disenfranchisement as Empathic Failure: Grief Therapy and the Co-Construction of Meaning." In Kenneth Doka, ed., *Disenfranchised Grief: New Directions, Challenges, and Strategies for Practice* (Champaign, Illinois: Research Press, 2002): 95–118.

15. Thomas Attig, "Respecting Bereaved Children and Adolescents," *Beyond the Innocence of Childhood (Volume 3): Helping Children and Adolescents Cope with Death and Bereavement,* ed., David Adams and Eleanor DeVeau (Amityville, New York: Baywood Press, 1995).

16. Thomas Attig, "Beyond Pain: The Existential Suffering of Children," *Journal of Palliative Care* xx (1996): xx–yy.

17. Thomas Attig, "Respecting the Spirituality of the Dying and the Bereaved," *A Challenge for Living: Dying, Death, and Bereavement,* ed., Inge Corless, Barbara Germino and Pittman-Lindeman (New York: Jones and Bartlett, 1995). Revised as "Respecting the Spiritual Beliefs of the Dying and the Bereaved" for inclusion in the Second Edition (2002).

18. Martin Heidegger, *Being and Time*, trans. John Macquarrie and James M. Robinson (New York: Harper & Row, 1962).

19. Thomas Attig, "Questionable Assumptions about Assumptive Worlds," in *Loss of the Assumptive World: A Theory of Traumatic Loss*, ed., Jeffrey Kaufman (Washington, D.C.:Bruner-Routledge, 2002).

20. See chapter 2 for a critique of the currently most well-known description (in J. William Worden's writings) of grieving in terms of these dimensions of living and grief work as "tasks" when they most assuredly are no such thing. The critique there of the first and second editions of his book, *Grief Counseling and Grief Therapy: A Handbook for the Mental Health Practitioner* (New York: Springer 1982 and 1991) still apply to the recently released fourth edition (2009).

21. Thomas Attig, "Relearning the World: Making and Finding Meanings," in *Meaning Reconstruction and the Experience of Loss*, ed. Robert Neimeyer (Washington, D.C., American Psychological Association, 2001).

22. Margaret Stroebe and Henk Schut, "The Dual-Process Model of Coping with Bereavement: Rationale and Description," *Death Studies* 23 (1999): 197–224.

23. Thomas Attig, *The Heart of Grief: Death and the Search for Lasting Love* (New York: Oxford University Press, 2000).

24. George A. Bonannos, "Loss, Trauma, and Human Resilience," *American Psychologist* 59 (2004): 20–28 and Irwin Sandler, Sharlene Wolchik, and Tim Ayers, "Resilience Rather than Recovery: A Contextual Framework on Adaptation Following Bereavement," *Death Studies* 32 (2008): 39–73.

25. Thomas Attig, *The Heart of Grief*.

26. Dennis Klass, Phyllis Silverman, and Steven Nickman, eds., *Continuing Bonds: New Understandings of Grief* (Washington, D.C., Taylor and Francis, 1996).

27. Robert Neimeyer, "Constructivist Therapy," Video (Washington, D.C., American Psychological Association, 2004).

28. Thomas Attig "Anticipating the Transition to Loving in Absence," in *Clinical Dimensions of Anticipatory Mourning: Theory and Practice in Working with the Dying, Their Loved Ones, and Their Caregivers*, ed. Therese Rando (Champaign, Illinois: Research Press, 2000): 115–133.

How We Grieve

1

Stories of Grieving:
Listening and Responding

Martin and Louise

Myra, a seventy-eight-year-old woman, dies in a nursing home after a long struggle with multiple sclerosis. She had been admitted to the home only two years earlier when her caregivers at home became physically and psychologically exhausted and reluctantly saw no other alternative. Her partially demented husband, Fred, her children, Martin and Louise, and her five grandchildren, ranging in age from five to twenty-three, survive her. Nursing home personnel wonder how to bring the news to Fred and how to support him in his grief. Martin and Louise sigh in relief that Myra's long agony is over, yet long for her return, Louise far more intensely than Martin. Martin feels more responsible than ever for their father, yet both Martin and Louise feel childlike, as if their parents had abandoned them. The grandchildren need them, yet their own grief makes it hard for them to attend to the children's needs. As adult children who saw Myra's inevitable death coming, they sense that others expect them to "handle it" easily. Consequently, although they feel acutely the need for support from others, they admit this to no one. The grandchildren hurt in their own ways, some grieving for the first time and others confused by the responses of their bereaved parents and siblings.

Jennifer

Nineteen-year-old Jennifer gives birth to a stillborn baby. She feels helpless, ashamed, and terribly alone. She has never known such pain. While she is in the recovery room, her well-intentioned parents, John and Denise, attempt to arrange with a funeral director an immediate and quiet disposition of the body. Feeling helpless and somewhat ashamed themselves, they hope to protect their Jennifer from more difficult experiences and painful choices. The funeral director resists. He risks the ire of John and Denise but insists that Jennifer is competent to give direction to her own experiences. He believes that he would be guilty of professional malpractice were he to fail to solicit her wishes directly. He insists she has a right to see the baby if she wishes, to name it, and to participate in planning for disposition of the body.

Bill, Diane, and Margaret

Bill and Diane, in their late twenties, are stunned by a telephone call while on a second honeymoon, a weekend vacation. They had left their three children, Ann, Mike, and Jimmy, with Diane's sister and closest confidant, Mary, who had agreed to stay with the children in their own home so that their parents' unusual, brief absence would not disturb them. The call brought the terrible news that all four had died, while sleeping, of asphyxiation caused by a gas leak. On hearing the news, Bill pounds his head on the wall and Diane melts into uncontrollable sobbing. They cannot believe what they have heard until they see for themselves. The multiple losses are nearly too much to bear; they had been playing in a distant place when the four died. The prospect of returning to the home where so many died daunts them. Although they have always planned a large family, it will be some time before it is possible even to make love, much less contemplate having children again. Indeed, the future is nearly entirely clouded as they experience themselves as deprived of their purpose in living. The women's mother, Margaret, discovered the bodies after trying unsuccessfully to reach Mary by phone in the early morning (when the children usually watched cartoons on TV). Margaret has seen too much. She turns to her husband, Earl, for support, and he tells her that the best thing is to try to forget. She does not press him further both because he is a stubborn man and because she fears that he is susceptible to a second, and possibly fatal, heart attack. She does not sleep for months.

Ed, Elise, and David

Bobby, age six, dies unexpectedly in an emergency room of gunshot wounds to the abdomen. His parents, Ed and Elise, bring him there after he had removed his father's pistol from a nightstand while playing with a friend, David. The weapon accidentally discharged as he handled it. Ed's guilt crushes him. Attempts to distract himself at work are unavailing. Elise's anger lingers barely beneath the surface, and she suffers from repeated and prolonged bouts of uncontrollable weeping. Both parents hold their feelings in out of fear of losing each other and thereby compounding their losses. Neither Ed nor Elise can fathom the meaning of the seemingly pointless death of a child so bright with promise. Bobby's brother and sister, Johnny and Melanie, who had seen him playing with the gun previously and said nothing to their parents, silently wish that the nightmare would end and Bobby revive. The grandparents, who had lectured Ed about the dangers of keeping the gun in the house, cannot console him. David is in shock, given what he has witnessed. His parents, Bruce and Barbara, seek professional help for him for his persistent nightmares, excessive clinging to them, and refusal to return to school. They worry about the long-term effects of this early traumatic experience.

Kathryn

Mark, thirty-eight years old, dies of an inoperable brain tumor, and his wife, Kathryn (a nurse), and his two children, Josh, age 5, and Sarah, age 3 survive him. Although the couple anticipated Mark's death, putting their financial house in order and completing a living will, and planned for life after he died (including career development for Kathryn and even possible remarriage), the death nevertheless devastates Kathryn. She and Mark always cooperated extensively and wonderfully in parenting the children. Constructing an independent life, with her children dependent on her now more than ever, presents many challenges. She faces possible physical and emotional overload in meeting both her own needs and those of the children. In her pain and anguish, Kathryn searches for the resources to see her through her loneliness and the hard choices and difficult years ahead. She wonders about the fairness of Mark's life ending so early and her children's facing a future without a father and about her own capacities to carry on without him. She finds consolation in prayer and refuses to allow her love for Mark to die along with him. Kathryn vows that her children will know who their father was and regularly tells them stories about episodes in his life. The death transforms Josh's and Sarah's lives, too, and they undoubtedly will miss Mark at virtually all key points in their personal development.

Colleen

A single woman, Sheila, twenty-eight, kills herself, writes no suicide note, and leaves family and friends with the mystery of her motivations. Her parents, Colleen and Jack, divorced when she was a teenager. Although Sheila lived with her mother, she became seriously estranged from her before escaping to college in a distant state. Hesitant reconciliation began only about a year before Sheila's suicide. Sheila's survivors search their souls for the means of understanding the tragic action, and each struggles to reconcile a love for her with hatred for what she has done. Most are uncomfortably silent about Sheila and her death. The sudden and unexpected disruption in their lives embarrasses some who are bothered by the social stigma of suicide, prompts others to resent the apparent selfishness of the act, and tempts still others to pretend that the death was accidental. Colleen alone pursues greater understanding of Sheila's life and death by seeking out the friends who knew her in her last years. As she does so, she struggles to understand and forgive herself. She is especially torn by her belief that suicide is an unforgivable sin, and she seeks greater understanding and consolation in prayer.

Stories Are the Heart of the Matter

I am well acquainted with stories like those I have just presented.[1] Most of us have experienced similar loss. Some of us may recognize a family member, a friend, or ourselves among the people I describe here. Stories like these never fail to move me, and when I hear them I want to offer support. My listening by itself is helpful, but I want to do more. Those who tell their stories appreciate an attentive, patient listener and long for more in response. They want to be understood *and* to be supported as they come to terms with what has happened to them.

Stories shared with me over the years ground my reflections throughout this book. I hope these reflections are faithful to the stories and provide keys to understanding persons who lose someone through death. I hope too that the ideas here motivate readers to listen carefully to those who have suffered loss and suggest ways of supporting those whose stories they hear.

Each person mentioned in the previous pages has a life story to tell. Part of what it is to be a person is to embody such a life story. No biography replicates any other. To understand these persons as individuals, you must learn the details of each life story and how each person finds identity as those details unfold. Losses through death hold a unique place in each survivor's life story. When losses occur, individuals and their experiences do not suddenly fit some preordained pattern. No story of loss replicates any other. To understand any one of the experiences of loss I have sketched, you must learn the details of the story each survivor has to tell about how the loss has changed profoundly his or her experience of the world and has limited what is possible in the next chapters of each biography. You must learn the different ways the death disrupts the flow of each survivor's life story. You must learn how each survivor faces distinct challenges and struggles to go on in the next chapters of life.

I flesh out each of the stories sketched here in greater detail in the chapters that follow. I do so, in part, to illustrate some of the diversity of experiences of loss through death. I cannot, and do not, pretend to be comprehensive in capturing the limitless variety of possible loss and coping experiences. I strive only to be representative.

I also elaborate on these stories to sustain focus where I believe it belongs—that is, on the poignancy of disruption of life entailed by loss and on the daunting challenges persons address as they cope. In treating concrete, vivid, personal accounts prominently, I reverse the usual emphasis in developing ideas about loss and coping. Writers and speakers commonly emphasize their ideas and treat stories as merely anecdotal. I believe that stories of loss through death are the heart of the matter in reflection on loss and coping. As I see it, the point of developing any ideas on the subject is to foster better understanding of, and more effective response to, individuals living with loss. I believe that the most important test of the worth of the ideas I develop is whether they enhance understanding of individual stories. I regularly introduce new ideas through storytelling to show how the ideas do such service. I hope these ideas can serve as keys to understanding how specific losses disrupt individual biographies. Thus I will develop general ideas about coping with loss only insofar as the ideas can serve as keys to understanding how coping changes the course of particular lives. I will develop general ideas about effective means of supporting persons as they cope with loss only insofar as the ideas can serve to shape effective support for individuals struggling with challenges uniquely their own. At best, the ideas I develop can in these ways ease entrance into dialogue with the individuals we care about and hope to comfort or serve as prelude to understanding our own loss experiences and coping needs.

Bereavement, Grieving, and Mourning Defined

I have thus far avoided the use of any technical vocabulary, and I intend to use it only minimally, defining terms as I go. I could hardly write this book without clarifying how I intend to use three key terms: bereavement, grief, and mourning.

I use the term *bereavement* to refer to the state or condition caused by loss through death. When any of us loses someone we care about, we are deprived of their companionship. The deprivation is, by definition, bereavement. Having been so deprived, we are bereaved persons. When we are bereaved, the world presents a different environment in which we must live, one where the palpable absence of the other pervades, we anguish, our present lives are thrown into disarray, and the flow of our life stories is disrupted. Bereavement redefines and limits our life possibilities.

Writings on *grieving* and *mourning* define the terms variously and sometimes ambiguously. Without an extensive defense of my choices, I intend to use the terms *grieving* and *mourning* to refer to processes of accommodating to loss. Grieving and mourning are coping responses to the deprivation and disruption that enter our lives when we are bereaved. As we grieve and mourn, we address our new life situation, come to terms with the absence of the one who has died, deal with our anguish, pick up the pieces of our shattered lives, and move into the next chapters of our biographies which are indelibly colored by our bereavement.

I use *mourning* in two different ways. On the one hand, *mourning* refers to what we do within ourselves to transform our relationship to the one who has died. When we have cared about persons when they were present, what happens to our caring now that they are gone? Can we still care, only in a different way? As we search for ways of living with answers to these questions, we mourn. On the other hand, *mourning* refers to the ways our societies and cultures tell us to behave in response to loss through death, including prescribed practices in the funeral period and, in some cultures, for a year or more thereafter. Societies and cultures establish such mourning practices to provide stabilizing expectations and behaviors for us during a time that we often experience as confusing and chaotic. The practices also enable others to readily recognize us as bereaved, tolerate our emotions and actions more easily, and support us during the prescribed period.

In contrast, I use *grieving* to refer to the full range of our coping responses to loss through death, including, but not confined to, socially defined mourning practices, or what we do within ourselves to redefine our relationship with the deceased. I also use *grieving* to refer to our coping response to any significant loss experiences, such as when we divorce, lose a friendship, lose a home, lose a job, or suffer physical disabilities or amputations (though not when we lose such things as small wagers or a toothbrush). I use *mourning*, however, to refer only to responses to loss through death. Although the ideas about grieving that I develop in this book can be usefully extended (albeit at times with important modification) to illuminate the broader range of loss experiences, I focus on grieving following death.

I enter but one caution. In Chapter 2 I develop a further distinction between grief as a specific emotion and grieving as a coping process. We experience the emotion grief as we notice the absence of the deceased and long for his or her return. Grief is a part of the anguish aroused in us in bereavement. I use the term *grief*, then, to refer both to this emotion and to the process of coping. (I use the term *mourning* in a similarly ambiguous way in that when we feel the emotion grief we are said in doing so to mourn.) In Chapter 2 I argue that effective coping with loss requires that we resist the temptation to dwell in a potentially paralyzing state of extreme grief.

Why Do People Look to Books on Grieving?

Many, if not most, of the persons who share their stories of bereavement and grieving tell me that they looked for books or speeches about what they are experiencing. Many who wish to comfort and support the bereaved also turn to such sources. These searches frequently end in disappointment. I have listened carefully to such search stories and found that some seekers know precisely what they want from such sources, while others have but the vaguest ideas of what they want. I have learned much about what disappoints them and about the perspectives, ideas, insights, and guidance they seek. In the chapters that follow, I do what I can to offer a better response to these needs. But first, how can we understand what these needs are?

They Seek General Understanding

Martin and Louise, like so many others I have met, feel isolated and alone in their grieving. They wonder whether anyone understands what it is like for them. Their bereavement is unprecedented in their experiences, and they long for reassurance that they are not living in a world that has no idea of what they are going through. Some survivors, like Martin and Louise, feel the need for support from others but admit it to no one for fear of being misunderstood. Many others tell me that others say such foolish and inappropriate things that it is clear that they have little useful understanding to offer.

As they turn to books in privacy, mourners frequently seek reassurance in perceptive and sympathetic *general understanding from others*. Some hope to find a book that they can give to others who seem to understand so little of their anguish and struggle; many who want to offer comfort and support also turn to books to find ways to understand better those they care about in a time of need.

Too often, mourners find authors whose ideas simply fail to resonate with their experiences. They don't recognize themselves, what has befallen them, or their struggles in what is being said. Theoretical books on grieving fail to capture the principal shape and substance of what it has been like for them to lose and now to have to go on. The writings seem cold, impersonal, analytic, and distant. The descriptions and generalizations seem off the mark. Some authors write of predictable sequences of experience that all persons go through, but to the bereaved there seems to be no order in their lives at all. Others write as if there were something wrong with, even pathological, about the bereaved as they struggle with something that surely enters each of our lives eventually. Can it really be somehow abnormal to grieve if everyone does it? This kind of thinking simply does not ring true to most people I have talked to. Infact, encounters with these writings put many people off, and they begin to think that there may be no reassuring understanding of grieving to be found anywhere. Moreover, they are put off by others in their lives who read those same books or harbor similar theories and seek to impose on them an understanding that just does not fit.

Other mourners turn to the countless first-person accounts of grieving. Here they find warmth and someone who has been through a similar experience. Still, the writings concentrate on the details of the authors' own distinct experiences and expose readers to pain in addition to their own. Often it is as if the reader were in that all too typical conversation with another who hopes to be helpful but instead diverts attention to, and then dwells on, personal loss rather than speaking to the grieving person's loss. Readers may find reassurance that they are not the only ones who grieve, but they do not find either sympathy or the reassurance that they are understood by others. When such authors offer a general perspective on grieving, it is so often colored by their own personal experience or influenced by familiar theories that it, too, fails to resonate with the mourner's experience.

To respond to the shortcomings of other theoretical and personal approaches to grieving, I offer the idea of grieving as a process of relearning the world, which I believe captures the broad spectrum of experiences associated with grieving. Martin and Louise learned their own ways of being in the world prior to Myra's death. Their bereavement disrupts the pattern of living they have learned, and as they grieve they learn new ways. So, too, with the rest of us. Mourners should find the stabilizing reassurance they seek here in descriptions that resonate with their experiences. Those who would comfort and support them should find the means to understand what those they care about are experiencing. My generalizations should not be expected to capture the central features of, or the essence of, every possible grieving experience.[2] While each of us relearns in our own way, I describe the common threads and family resemblances among our ways of doing so.

Jennifer, like so many other mourners I have spoken with, longs for people who will understand her. It would comfort her to know that family and friends appreciate what has happened to her and what she struggles with. Unfortunately, although grieving is among the most widely shared human experiences, its general character is not well understood. It pains Jennifer that only her funeral director, Terry, seems to have an inkling of what she faces and how much it hurts. Why don't the others know? Beyond reassurance that some author who is a stranger to them understands, mourners hope to find ideas that could help intimates to understand them better. Everyone who wishes to empathize with, and respond appropriately to, the bereaved needs a way of going about it, and so many seek a useful framework in books. Readers (mourners and those who wish to comfort them as well) become discouraged when they find discussions of grieving that seem intended only for a select few, be they scientific researchers, scholars, or highly trained professionals.[3] It does not seem reasonable to them to describe such a universal human experience in technical and obscure terms. Given that loss through death touches everyone and that most persons are at some time motivated to reach out and help others who grieve, it seems reasonable to hope for, and expect, ideas that are intelligent and yet *broadly accessible*.

I believe that my idea of grieving as a process of relearning the world is readily accessible to all. This book explores this idea throughout it discussions. I first sketch prominent, and all too familiar, metaphors and analogies in other writing about grieving (predominantly social scientific, clinical, and personal accounts)[4] and show how the idea of relearning the world idea has great advantages. Grieving is an elusive and opaque subject to most of us. However, learning one's way in the world is familiar, or can be made easily accessible, to reflective readers. From a broadly accessible discussion of how we find our bearings in the world, it is a short leap to seeing how bereavement disrupts the process of learning our way in the world demanding we learn new ways of going on without those who have died. I hope to show how grieving is such a relearning process and, in so doing, shed light on the obscure by relating it to what is familiar and better or more easily understood.[5]

Although understanding from others is something that Bill and Diane desperately want and need, it is not sufficient. They also seek, perhaps most importantly, *self-understanding*. The deaths of their three children, Ann, Mike, and Jimmy, together with that of Diane's sister Mary make a shambles of Bill's and Diane's lives. These terrible events confuse and disorient them profoundly. They feel as if their lives are shattered. The world has dealt them cruel blows in every facet of their being. The deaths bring emotional turmoil and shake their self-confidence. They doubt their worthiness as parents, and they wonder who they are, given what has happened to them. Are they still their children's mother and father? Daily living was filled with and devoted to the children. Those patterns of living now make no sense, and the long days seem empty, devoid of purpose. Intense emotion and unceasing tension and strain leave them on the brink of exhaustion, and they sense that physical breakdown could come. Their children's and sister's absences are palpable as Bill and Diane long to see, hold, touch, and kiss them and to be seen, held, touched, and kissed in return. The ache of separation is with them constantly and unlike anything they have ever felt. How strange it is to be with each other and their fellow survivors, especially Margaret and Earl. Both are in new and different places since the deaths (reminiscent of Munch's *Death Chamber*). The deaths strain, even threaten to break, virtually all their connections with others, including family, friends, and those at work. Everything that has happened seems so senseless. Their heads swim with questions. How did this happen? Did they suffer? Why must children die? What can life mean when it ends so prematurely? What does any life mean anyway? The new life landscape in which they must live is radically different from the one that preceded it. It presents challenges that are too numerous to count, unsorted and tangled, and that seem to press upon them all at once. The weight of the new world threatens to overwhelm them. They have no idea whether they can put their lives back together again. How is it possible to do so, and where are they to begin? They recognize that their lives can never be the same, and they wonder if it can be worth it to continue living. Just how life could be good and meaningful again lies beyond their reckoning as they struggle to go on in a pervasive agony.

Like Bill and Diane, mourners turn to books for a self-understanding that allows them to see their experiences of loss within a general framework. Useful ideas enable them to sort out just what has happened to them, to understand the challenges before them, and to learn what can come from meeting those challenges in a future new and inevitably different from the one they had anticipated prior to bereavement. They search for ideas that acknowledge how bereavement and grieving enter, change, and pervade their lives. They experience the impact of their losses in all facets of their lives: the emotional and psychological, the behavioral, the biological and physical, the social, and the intellectual and spiritual. Bereavement affects whole persons. In turn, grieving persons must cope with loss in all of these same facets of their lives. Whole persons grieve. Finally, the changes affected through coping (successful or unsuccessful) tend to be pervasive and life-transforming. Whole persons become different through loss and grieving. It is tempting to concentrate on one facet of grieving at a time, but to do so misses the pervasiveness of the experience and courts the danger of mistaking a part for the whole. For example, psychodynamic, behaviorist, biological attachment, family systems, and rational/cognitive writings about grieving distort the phenomena and, consequently, make it difficult for readers to gain self-understanding of the whole of what they experience as they grieve.

My idea of grieving as relearning the world responds to these needs as well. Learning our way in the world and then relearning when we are bereaved is not simply a cognitive matter of mastering ideas; it is not a matter of learning *that* the world is different because someone we care about has died. Instead, the learning and relearning involve investment of ourselves as whole persons, in all facets of our life all at once, as we learn *how* to be ourselves in the world before, and then relearn after someone we care about dies. Through such relearning we find and make ways of living with our emotions and struggle to reestablish self-confidence, self-esteem, and identity in a biography colored by loss. We strive to adapt our behaviors and daily life patterns to new life circumstances not of our own choosing and to recover our sense of daily purpose. We seek means of meeting our physical and biological needs (including our need for closeness with others). We seek ways of being with fellow survivors and to connect meaningfully once again with others at home, within our families, with friends, at work, and in the world at large. We search for answers to questions about what has happened, and we seek to place the death and our lives in a context of belief that enables us to renew hope and to find consolation, peace, and meaning as we go on living.

As she grieves for her daughter Sheila, Colleen is greatly impatient with others, especially her former husband, Jack, who insists that she "will get over it in time." She senses vaguely that she may never do so. And it strikes her as unseemly to suggest that she will or should. It seems to her that coming to terms with Sheila's unexpected and tragic suicide will be a struggle to which she will return again and again throughout her remaining days. She senses that she will not settle in one place once and for all in coming to terms with her daughter's death. She learned from the years when Sheila was alive that life flows unpredictably. Before the divorce, life with Sheila was good. Then came the turmoil, Sheila's rebellion, and their estrangement after the divorce. Just as mother and daughter were making progress in reconciliation, Sheila killed herself. These experiences humble Colleen. She has learned to expect the unexpected and to take one step at a time on what now seems a life's journey that ever eludes her firm control and where what is done is often painfully undone.

Kathryn, having anticipated and discussed openly with Mark his death and her widowhood, is determined not to be undone by the loss. Yet she senses that the challenges she faces are unlike any others she has known. She is startled to find that anticipation of Mark's death did not prepare her for the shattering effects of bereavement. His death could not be neatly packaged and handled in advance, even through detailed planning. Addressing the challenges feels vaguely different from anything she has every done before, though words to describe what it is like escape her. She muses that it is as if she and Mark had treated his death, and her life after it, as a large puzzle that they could solve together and in advance. But now there seem an infinite number of pieces, and there is no way of telling how, or if, they fit together. Putting some pieces together provides temporary stability and comfort, but new pieces are always being added presenting new challenges as the unfinished "puzzle" changes shape almost daily. She finds and then loses stability and comfort over and over again. She realizes how little control she has over events in her life as she does what she can to find a way of going on. In prayer she finds trust, even without complete control, and although clear direction eludes her now, there is a way. She braces for more surprises and anticipates that she and her children, Josh and Sarah, will be coming to terms with Mark's death as long as they live.

The stories of Colleen and Kathryn illustrate what is perhaps most unsettling yet most fascinating about grieving—that *mystery* pervades our human condition. Mourners like Colleen and Kathryn need to recognize, and others who comfort them must also recognize, that the bereaved are dealing not with ordinary, day-to-day problems but rather with mystery as they struggle to come to terms with loss through death. Mourners are put off by others who fail to see how the shape and proportion of what lies before them is anything but ordinary and who offer simple advice about what they need to do to address their losses. They rightly set aside books that give no hint of understanding how daunting their situation is, and they reject those who try to comfort them by parroting superficial words of understanding. Grieving reminds them, and us, of the profundity, of the mystery of living an individual life, in which struggles with finiteness, change, uncertainty, and vulnerability recur and persist.

Mysteries, and not simply problems, hold center stage in our lives when we grieve. This is what Colleen, Kathryn, and others sense when they feel that bereavement presents challenges unlike others they have faced. Problems are challenges that we can solve, answer definitively, control, manage, or master. We can find satisfactory resolution for problems and move on. Mysteries, in contrast, present challenges that we cannot deal with so decisively. Because of this, as we relearn the world in grieving we do not simply solve problems. Mysteries are ever-present elements of our surroundings, conditions of ongoing living that are too important for us to ignore and that yet persistently challenge and provoke us. We cannot overcome the mysteries or dissipate the challenges that they represent by solving or resolving them. We have no choice but to confront these enigmas again and again, to come to terms with or learn to live with them as they command our attention in some of the most difficult times of our lives. Mysteries present themselves in ever-changing perspectives that reveal ever-new facets and that transcend our understanding or our ability to cope with them definitively. I believe that we relearn the world in grieving again and again throughout our lives as we learn an acceptable way of going on for a time and then find that we must change course once again. As we encounter mysteries, we must learn and relearn to let go and resist the temptation of believing that they are ultimately solvable, manageable, controllable, or manipulable.

Mysteries make the limits of our ideas transparent. We must see that even the most appropriate ideas and the most acutely perceptive understanding of the realities of death and suffering cannot change them. They remain unperturbed. Only we can change in response to them. Although our thinking cannot change them, we can define, individually and collectively, appropriate coping responses. Despite a fundamental limitation of our ideas, there remains an enduring point to doing the best we can in finding our way through even our most difficult experiences, in struggling to relearn. Some paths are better than others in coping with loss and relearning the world. But not all persons are suited to the same paths, and not all find their way. Ultimately, the mysteries remain beyond our grasp or control.

They Seek Respect for Individuality

Ed and Elise, as they grieve for their little Bobby, cringe when others say (as they far too often do) "I know how you feel" or "I know what it must be like for you." How could anyone presume to know any such thing? The audacity of others who pretend to know what life is like for them awes them, and they resent it deeply. Others who have lost a child understand some of what it's like, and they have the good sense not to speak so foolishly. Who knows what it was like to decide to bring Bobby into the world? Who else could know what it was like to struggle through those early nights of his infancy, delight as they watched him grow and play, celebrate every "first" with him, share in his daily adventures, close the day with a story and tuck him into bed, nurse him when he was ill, know so well what made him laugh, feel his arms about their necks or the warmth of his kisses? Who else could know what it was like to discover what he had done that terrible day, hold him in their arms on the way to the hospital, or wait helplessly through those long minutes that seemed like hours, only to hear, "We're sorry. We did all we could"? How could anyone know what it is like to face what they now face: the gun, their own bedroom, the site of the accident, each other's emotional turmoil, Bobby's older brother and sister, their neighbors and their little boy, David, who was there when it happened? Ed and Elise find it impossible to talk candidly with one another about what they have been through. They long fervently for someone who will listen patiently to the details of their stories of life with Bobby, the events surrounding his death, and their lives in the days since. They sense that telling these things will itself help them to begin to deal with what has happened—if they could only find someone who recognizes how much the details matter to them.

For Ed and Elise, as for virtually all the grieving persons who have shared their stories with me, for others to have a general understanding of grieving is not enough. Yes, it allays their fears that they are not alone in grief. Beyond this, however, they want understanding and *respect as individuals and for the uniqueness of their experiences.* Whatever can be said about grieving persons in general (or even about grieving men or women, spouses, mothers or fathers, or other categories of mourners) can only scratch the surface of these unprecedented experiences. Respect requires appreciation of how the death has disrupted the survivors' biographies in their unique life circumstances and how they confront specific, concrete challenges as they move into the next chapters of their life stories.[6] When mourners turn to books for understanding, they often grow impatient with discussions that seem to reduce the experiences of all who grieve to the lowest common denominator, as if somehow all loss experiences were remarkably homogeneous. They resent authors who write as if what can be said in general is enough, as if statistics tell the most important story, and who treat stories of particular grieving persons as incidental. Ideas about the general contours of grieving inevitably describe incompletely and fail to capture the detail, subtlety, and nuance of individual experiences. As flesh-and-blood individuals mourners live and anguish in those details. Only in the details can they and their grief be understood. Good ideas provide clues as to what to look for in becoming acquainted with and responding respectfully and sensitively to the all-important particulars of stories of loss that bereaved persons have to tell.

The idea of grieving as relearning the world is ideally suited to serve mourners and those who would understand them in this way. No two of us learn an identical way of being our own person and living in the world. No two of us experience the same disruption in our life story. No two of us confront the same challenges in facing the future. And no two of us will relearn the same way of being ourselves or living the next chapters of our lives. The general account of the relearning that I develop in later chapters provides the kind of framework for dialogue and respect for individuals that mourners seek. I show how we relearn as whole persons in all facets of our lives, and as I do so, I encourage dialogue in which listeners can hear the details of the emotional and psychological, behavioral, physical, social, and intellectual and spiritual challenges that particular grieving persons face. I describe the general contours of the world that we inhabit, including our physical surroundings and our place in the larger scheme of things, our social surroundings (including the deceased and, for some, the divine), and ourselves at the centers of unique experiences of the world. As I do so, I encourage dialogue about which concrete and specific elements or aspects of each person's distinctive surroundings or unique self are most challenging.

They Seek Ways to Deal with Helplessness in Grieving

When Jennifer loses her stillborn baby boy, when Margaret loses her daughter Mary and her three grandchildren, they feel powerless and helpless. Jennifer carried her baby to term, yet was deprived of ever knowing his personality or being loved as his mother. She feels as if she has been cheated by forces beyond her understanding. Margaret's losses crash into her life with devastating power. She, too, feels robbed by a seemingly arbitrary and cruel event. Each is acutely aware that she had no control whatever over what has befallen her, no choice in this defining moment in her life. Each feels small and insignificant in the face of these overwhelming events, as if she were at the mercy of a chaotic universe. Their feelings of powerlessness and helplessness paralyze them. They wonder whether there is any room for control in their lives. They are at a loss as to what to do or say that can possibly make any difference. Fortunately for Jennifer, her funeral director understands such helplessness. He presents options to her and shows her that she has choice about how she responds to her son's death and how she can give direction to her life in its aftermath. Unfortunately, Margaret does not find such support early in her bereavement, and she walks the floor alone at night in anguish and despair.

When bereavement and its devastating effects enter our lives, we often feel powerless and helpless. Death is such a choiceless event; it is something that happens to those we care about, and we have little or no control over it. Similarly, we have no choice about the havoc that death brings into our daily lives and the disruption of our life stories that it entails. The resultant chaos and disorder so pervade the landscape that many of us begin to suspect that the possibility of control in life is an illusion. Often when the bereaved turn to books they search for ideas about what they themselves can do and say in their new and difficult circumstances. They seek ideas that will restore their confidence that they have meaningful choice and that they can somehow find their way onto a new and once again meaningful life path. Unfortunately, the ideas in many books reinforce their feelings of powerlessness and helplessness. Grieving is often discussed as something that happens to people, something that they must endure passively. Or it is discussed in terms of unconscious or preconscious dimensions of their experiences over which people have no choice or control.[7] Or grieving is discussed in a language so inaccessible that it leaves the impression that understanding and dealing with grief is in the hands of a few scientists or professionals who pretend to know better how to give direction to the lives of survivors.[8] Grieving persons need to hear that as we grieve we cope actively. Although bereavement happens to us, grieving is what we do in response to it. Far from being choiceless, our coping is pervaded by choice.[9]

My ideas about grieving as relearning the world are responsive to mourners' feelings of powerlessness and helplessness. Bereavement jolts us off the path we have learned to follow in life and leaves our lives in disarray. As we relearn our ways of being in the world, we identify, explore, test, and ultimately appropriate new ways of going on. As we relearn how to be in a world that is drastically changed by what has happened, we always have options in how we meet the emotional and psychological, behavioral, physical, social, and intellectual and spiritual challenges we face. We can choose our own responses to the things and places left behind and to our fellow survivors, the deceased, and even God. We can choose how we reshape our daily lives, reinterpret and redirect our life stories, and find our way back to purposeful, meaningful, and hopeful life again. Such are the basic contours of relearning the worlds of our experience. Understanding these things can itself support mourners in sorting their own needs, options, and preferences and enable them to take charge of defining the next chapters of their lives. It gives them concrete ideas about what to do and say as they address the challenges before them. Among these things is to communicate more effectively about what their grieving involves and what might be helpful to those who would support and comfort them.

They Seek Guidance for Caregivers

Each of the mourners in the stories has difficulty in finding comfort and support from others. Martin and Louise are barely recognized in their grieving. Family and friends seem to think that, as mature adults who long expected Myra's death, they should feel relief that she no longer suffers and therefore have little trouble in getting on with their lives. Martin and Louise feel in a way abandoned by those who care about them, and this feeling compounds the feeling (that they admit to no one) that they've been abandoned by their mother. The nursing home offered a one-day talk on grieving that they attended long before Myra died, but the generalities and pat formulas they heard there did not come close to capturing what they now experience or meeting their needs.

Jennifer's parents have good intentions as they try to do difficult things for her, but they fail to realize that only she can come to terms with what has happened to her. Their presumption feels to her like an attempt to control her life and adds to her feelings of alienation from them. Her friends, none of whom has ever been pregnant, have no clue about what she is going through, and as they avoid her or speak in empty clichés, they compound her feeling that she is alone in her grief. Fortunately, Terry, her funeral director, offers empathy and understanding of the challenges and choices she faces.

The devastation in Bill's and Diane's lives when their three children and sister die is of such a scale that it frightens many potential supporters away. Bill and Diane sense that some other parents and couples avoid them because they do not want to be reminded of what could happen to them. Bill's family simply does not talk about such difficult life events. Friends at Rotary tell Bill uselessly to "be strong" or "take good care of Diane," not recognizing how much he needs warm response. Those at work seem determined to go on with business as if nothing has happened. Diane's family is more receptive to her talking, but she misses being able to confide in her closest sister, Mary. Diane finds wives in other couples who will at least listen, though she misses being together as couples. Bill's and Diane's distance from Margaret, Diane's mother, who found the bodies, is rooted in her reluctance to tell them anything of what she saw or has experienced since and in their fear of her fragility and what they might hear. Margaret herself approaches her husband, Earl, only to be rebuffed with the painfully inadequate advice that "it's best just to forget it."

Ed and Elise receive little or no support from each other in the aftermath of Bobby's death. Ed's guilt and Elise's anger get in the way, and each feels terribly isolated. They hear nothing from their neighbors, Bruce and Barbara, who are furious at them for what their son, David, witnessed in their home. Elise's parents, who had cautioned Ed not to have the gun in the house, are no help at all as both couples avoid contact. Ed's friends and fellow workers are so far from understanding what it is like for him that their consoling remarks or platitudes would be laughable were they not so irritating. Fortunately, Elise finds warmth and empathy in a support group, though she wishes she didn't have to turn to strangers to find what she needs.

David's parents have no idea how to help him with his nightmares, his clinging to them, and his refusal to return to school. Though he says he wants to go to Bobby's funeral, Bruce and Barbara tell him that they think it best that he not be exposed to such a sad event. In part, they stay away because they do not want to confront Ed and Elise. Their instinct is to try to protect David. They understand well that David's troubles derive from his seeing his best friend shot in the house next door, but their holding him, drying his tears, keeping him at home seem not enough. Efforts to get him to talk about his experience don't work, it seems in part because he just does not have the words. They sense that David needs help that they don't know how to give, and they approach a counselor, who is able to give David the help he needs.

Kathryn experiences isolation from others as she spends much of her time tending to the needs of her children, Josh and Sarah. Before Mark died there was an outpouring of care and concern from relatives and friends. Now, so many seem to be hesitant to approach her. "They have such busy lives of their own," she thinks. "They just don't know what it's like living with this day after day and night after night." Only when she takes the initiative does she find that others will listen patiently and help her put her life back together. Still, it is so difficult to find a new place in the world as a single mother. The world seems made for couples. She finds solace and hope in prayer. She particularly enjoys "remember-when" sessions with her children. They seem so at ease with what the others deal with only reluctantly.

When Colleen's daughter Sheila commits suicide, Colleen notices the embarrassing silence that surrounds her. The death is literally unspeakable to so many in her family and among her friends. So many are embarrassed about what Sheila has done, and some even try to pretend that the death was an accident. "How," she wonders, "can anyone come to terms with this, or help me, if they aren't even going to acknowledge the reality of what Sheila has done?" She is frustrated that so many others refuse to discuss why Sheila did it or express any loving feelings about Sheila. Colleen is hit hard by her former husband seeming to blame her for what has happened, though she is not surprised. When she sets out to find answers and to learn more about Sheila's last years of life, she is actively discouraged by family and friends from doing what she feels she needs most to do.

When we mourn, we are often painfully aware of how difficult it is for others who care *about* us to find ways of caring *for* us. All too frequently our families and friends do not know what to do or say. Some people, who seem compelled to speak, utter empty platitudes or offer mindless advice. Others are reluctant to speak with or even to come to see us for fear of doing or saying the wrong thing. Still others seemingly cannot be bothered with either the awkwardness or the negative feelings they fear that meeting with us will arouse. This lack of understanding compounds our suffering as we experience distance and lack of empathy. In some instances family and friends become impatient or alienated and even withdrawn, which is even worse. Some of us turn to support groups or professionals, often hesitantly, for the care we need and want. Here, too, we are sometimes disappointed, since not all counselors are well acquainted with how bereavement challenges us or how we grieve in all facets of our lives. Even when we find what we search for in such places, the distance and the alienation from those closest to us still hurt as we return to daily life with family and friends.

Often grieving persons turn to books not only to find comfort for themselves but to help those who care about them to care better for them. And many who want to offer comfort and support recognize that they have little idea of what to do or say and turn to books for ideas about how to care for relatives and friends who grieve or about how to more effectively support their clients if they are professional caregivers. Unfortunately, many are disappointed as they find the kinds of failures of understanding I have already discussed at length. Most books that are truly helpful stop at urging that caregivers be available to and present with the bereaved, be patient, listen well without prejudice, and offer no unwelcome or inane advice. Rare, however, are constructive suggestions about how to support grieving persons as they address the many challenges they face. At the very least, mourners and their caregivers should reasonably expect ideas that promote understanding and that can help them overcome the distance that grows between the bereaved and the world around them. They seek grounds for empathy that will counter impatience, alienation, and the tendency to withdraw from the bereaved. They seek ideas about what to do and what to say that will be respectful, sensitive, and constructive. Grieving persons not only want and need a patient ear to hear what they have to tell; they want and need active listening that helps them to orient themselves and find ways of meeting the challenges they face. As they begin to actively address those challenges, they want and need support and comfort as they pick up the pieces of their shattered lives and enter the next chapters of their biographies.

The view of grieving as relearning the world provides fertile ground in which constructive guidance for caregivers can take root. Caregivers should resist any temptation to attempt to do the difficult work of coping for us when we are bereaved. Our coping with loss is a personal experience, as is all coping. No other person can grieve for us. The challenges are ours to meet; the choices are ours to make. Yet, there is much that others can do for us as we relearn our worlds, find new places in our physical and social surroundings, learn how to continue to care about those who have died in their absence,[10] and struggle to find new, meaningful, and hopeful direction for our life stories. Caregivers can help us to recognize the variety of psychological, behavioral, physical, social, intellectual, and spiritual challenges we face. They can help us to identify our options and effective means of addressing the particular challenges in our unique life circumstance. Caregivers can motivate and encourage us to actively engage in coping at our own pace and in ways that fit with who we have been and hope to be. They can support us in doing what we choose to do as they provide active listening, constructive feedback, direction or guidance, reassurance, companionship, and comfort as needed and appropriate. Caregivers can help us define and participate in the new daily life patterns we shape for ourselves. They can look to the future with us and help us decide where we want to go and how we want to get there. They can remain close and join us in the next chapters of our lives. Although the grieving is ours and ours alone to do, we need not grieve alone, and those who care about us can help us in all of these ways as we relearn our worlds.

Notes

1. The stories recounted here are composites of real-life stories. I have changed the details to protect the privacy of those whose stories I tell.

2. Indeed, I doubt that there are such things as essences (or clusters of invariable features) of any of the rich variety of experiences that we humans share.

3. There are legitimate purposes in scientific writings about grieving. I do not wish to dismiss the contributions of research scientists, especially psychologists, sociologists, biologists, and health-care professionals, since all of these researchers have advanced our understanding of grieving. My point here is that their writings are often not responsive to the needs of grieving persons or of those close to them, nor are they intended to be so.

This is so, I believe, because much scientific writing pursues a different purpose. Scientists focus on patterns in the experiences of populations of grieving persons and what can be learned about grieving in general from examining such populations Scientists are concerned fundamentally with explanation and prediction. Some want to explain and predict the impacts of bereavement, for example, after sudden, violent, or mutilating deaths as contrasted with deaths due to illness. Others seek understanding of what accounts for differences in coping capacities. Some want to explain or predict differences in the effectiveness of coping or support. Still others seek to account for differences in need for, or potential benefit from, limited support services. All of these, and others like them, are interesting and worthy research objectives.

However, it would be a mistake to construe scientific research as purely empirical data gathering. Scientists, too, work with guiding concepts as they develop and test hyphotheses. Because of this, they need ideas about grieving that both capture well the general contours of grieving and suggest new and fruitful lines of scientific research on loss and coping. Without adequate descriptions of the general character of grieving (the central phenomenon to be accounted for), any purported explanations or predictions would refer vaguely, not clearly. I hope that the more accurate descriptions of grieving that I develop in this book serve as a guiding idea for new research on loss and coping. I, however, do not pursue these scientific purposes here.

4. See the early sections of Chapter 2.

5. The sciences frequently and fruitfully use this strategy in the use of metaphors or analogies.

6. Later in this chapter and in a fuller treatment in Chapter 3 we explain how respect does not stop at such appreciation but also requires appropriately sensitive behaviors in response.

7. Much writing on attachment or bonding or on psychodynamics does this.

8. Much writing on psychodynamics, behaviorism, family systems, and rational-cognitive models of grieving does this.

9. Chapter 2 elaborates and defends this idea in detail.

10. See Chapter 6 for a detailed treatment of what is involved in this aspect of relearning.

2

Grieving Is Active:
We Need Not Be Helpless

What matters is not what life does
to you but rather what you do with
what life does to you.
                    Edgar Jackson

A ship is safe in harbor, but that is
not what a ship is for.
                    Thomas Aquinas

The Story of Martin and Louise

Myra's children, Martin and Louise, feel helpless after Myra's death at age seventy-eight in the nursing home. The loss revives the feelings of powerlessness they first knew when they learned of their mother's multiple sclerosis. Their frustration had grown steadily as they witnessed the long agony of Myra's slow decline over nearly three decades, the hated disease robbing them of the once vital, vibrant, patient, and gentle mother of their childhood. They so wanted to relieve her suffering but could not. Focused intently on her needs, they expected only relief when death came; the childlike feeling that their mother has abandoned them and the longing for her return now startle them. The feeling of abandonment reactivates little-acknowledged feelings of being neglected by their father, Fred, as he devoted increasingly more of his energy to caring for Myra. Given Fred's serious episodes of dementia, they dread both his suffering

See my "The Importance of Conceiving of Grieving as an Active Process," *Death Studies* (1991), for an earlier version of some of the thinking in this chapter.

after Myra's death and, later, having to watch a second slow parental decline. Moreover, they dread their own unprecedented grief and the new surprises it may bring.

In the last years that Myra and Fred were at home, Martin and Louise skewed their daily routines as they visited regularly and nearly exhausted their physical and psychological resources, not to mention the good wills of their spouses and children. Myra's worsening condition combined with Fred's advancing age made it impossible for Fred to carry the burdens alone. Then his dementia began, increasing markedly his dependence on others. Martin visited every evening after dining with his family, and he took responsibility for his parents' home maintenance and financial affairs. Louise often took her youngest daughter, Heather, now five, to spend the day with Myra and Fred and did nearly all of the cleaning and cooking. The greater time burden fell to Louise because she was not employed. Martin squeezed extra time from evenings and weekends, times that Louise had with her own family. Neither fully recognized the sacrifices made by the other. Neither voiced the resentment that each felt.

Myra's lingering illness and the onset of Fred's took their tolls on Martin and Louise, disrupted normal life patterns, and strained relations between them and with their spouses. Louise, especially, became nearly entirely absorbed with caring for her mother. Their spouses recognized Martin's and Louise's exhaustion and insisted that they take care of themselves. This led to the decision to place both parents in a nursing home, which Louise initially resisted. Even after the move, Martin and Louise spent much time and effort in their daily visits to the nursing home and continued to skew their daily routines. Martin did not know which was more draining: the earlier active caregiving or the later, far more passive, conversing and simply being with his parents. Louise continued to prepare food and bring it to the home despite the full menu provided there. She kept scissors handy to clip articles from papers and magazines to bring to her mother.

Changes in Myra's temperament as she deteriorated further strained relations within the family. It was hard to sense her appreciation for her children's sacrifices. The nursing home decision was one of the most difficult they had ever made. Louise's initial resistance complicated matters considerably. Myra rebuked them both bitterly about the decision, never really believing Louise's resistance sincere. Her words stung Martin and Louise (albeit differently) at the time and do so now in memory. They long to hear her words of forgiveness. Martin feels himself to have been the villain, and Louise feels herself the coward. They each said things they now regret and long to speak words of reconciliation. Martin wishes, and Louise aches, to reaffirm and show the love that each still feels for Myra. Although they realize she would be in agony if still alive, they nevertheless wish she were. Martin misses the cushion between him and his father. His yearning for Myra is episodic and wishful. Louise's desire for her return is at times nearly preoccupying. She fears she cannot go on without her mother.

Martin has become so accustomed to the routine built around his mother's illness that he now wonders what daily life will be like without that central focus. Louise has greater difficulty in believing her routine must end. Rather than the great relief they had expected with their release from the burdens of caring for their mother, they find the pressures to adjust nearly overwhelming.

Martin struggles to find words for the pain he experiences, including embarrassment at the persistent feelings of abandonment. He often catches himself as he is about to call the home to speak to Myra or begin his trips to the home expecting to see both of his parents when he arrives and when he occasionally drops her name in conversation as if she were still alive. Such incidents seem momentarily irrational to him, but he quickly shakes them off as painful reminders that Myra no longer lives and that he has much adjusting yet to do. Unaccustomed to asking for support, he approaches no one. Family, friends, and the nursing home staff seem not to recognize the hurt. Rather, they expect Martin to feel relieved, since his mother had suffered so and he had done so much to care for her.

Louise, too, cannot find words for her hurt. At times she senses that she has been abandoned, but at others she simply refuses to believe that Myra is gone. Unlike Martin, she does not simply catch herself starting to do what she used to do. Rather, she sometimes actually calls the home, only to be told again that Myra no longer lives there. She then bursts into tears and slams down the receiver. She continues to prepare food and cut clippings from the magazines and newspapers and takes them to the home. Only on her arrival does she realize that she cannot deliver them because she cannot find Myra. She sometimes leaves them with Fred, who doesn't realize that she expects him to share them with Myra. When Martin sees the clippings, he believes she brought them for his father. Louise is ambivalent about behaving as if Myra were still alive. Mostly, it feels good to continue in her old ways. But occasionally she senses that there is something "not right" about her behaviors, and she hopes no one notices them. Unaccustomed to asking for support, she too approaches no one. Family, friends, and the nursing home staff again fail to recognize the hurt and expect her to feel relieved of a tremendous burden.

The nursing home sponsored a one-hour talk on grief that Martin and Louise attended shortly after their parents entered the home. The speaker mentioned a number of stages of grieving that all persons must experience. The words, vaguely remembered, seem now entirely irrelevant and decidedly unhelpful. Martin expects that his grief will dissipate with time and that healing will come, but he cannot for the moment see how. He goes through the motions of daily life and makes small adjustments as he goes. Louise grieves more intensely and desperately, reeling before a seemingly relentless series of events beyond her control. She seriously doubts her pain will ever dissipate.

As they begin to live without Myra, Martin and Louise face many challenges. The very furniture of their lives challenges them daily; they own items given to them when Myra and Fred entered the nursing home, especially the parents' favorite recliner chairs. For now, Martin avoids his chair for the most part, although occasionally he sits in it and weeps. Louise, however, continues to sit in her mother's chair while cutting the clippings. And, of course, the pictures, scrapbooks, and other mementos present distinctive challenges to each. Martin's and Louise's relationships with their families are strained, sometimes greatly so, and complicated in that each family member is now grieving in his or her own way. Relationships with friends have long since been put on hold. Tensions between Martin and Louise linger and leave them uncomfortable even talking to each other. Both face spiritual crises. Martin wonders how the world, and ultimately God, can be so unfair and suffering seemingly unrelenting—first their mother, and now their father, with his growing incapacity. Just when Fred can have a life of his own, he has begun to lose his ability to live it. In his brighter moments, Martin feels the need for new balance in his daily routine, one without such singular devotion to parents and near-neglect of his own family. He seeks renewed purpose and hope for the future. In his darkest moments, he can't see the point of working and raising his family if it all comes to nothing better than this. His father's continuing need casts an ominous shadow. Still, he recognizes that his home life, especially his relationship with his wife, demands attention. By contrast, Louise's moments are mostly dark. Her intense longing for Myra's return distracts her from putting together a new life without her mother. She persists in the old pattern with her father and dreads what will come next. She doggedly continues her household routine with little sense of the growing impatience of her husband and children. She is too preoccupied in present longing to even think of renewed purpose and hope for the future. She desperately hopes that God will carry her and her mother and father through these awful times. The variety of challenges Martin and Louise face daunts them; Martin more than Louise senses the need to build a new life, but both doubt their own coping capacities.

Finally, Martin more than Louise recognizes that they are not alone as Myra's survivors. He sees Louise's intense and preoccupying distress, although he doesn't grasp the full extent of it, and he worries for her. He sees that Fred, too, is challenged by a world transformed by Myra's death. Most immediately, he wonders how Fred will be affected through the funeral period. He wonders how to support him then and over the long term as he learns to live without his companion of over fifty years. He worries especially about the implications of Fred's dementia for coping with the loss. He is at a loss as to what to do or say to help. Martin recognizes that his and Louise's own children are grieving, each in his or her own way. He is concerned about Louise's obvious inability to help her children but thinks it parallel to his own. He wonders how age affects grieving, and he worries particularly about the needs of the youngest, especially Louise's Heather, who was so close to her grandmother. He doesn't want the children to think the world is out of control but is tempted to think so himself. He wonders how to support the children through the funeral period and as they continue to grow. The children's questions challenge him, and he worries about the feelings that lay beneath the surface. He doubts his own abilities or energy to offer much support, at least in the short term, and reluctantly wonders whether others, perhaps his wife or brother-in-law, can help.

Jennifer's Story

Jennifer, too, feels helpless. Her loss revives the feelings of powerlessness she first knew when she learned of her pregnancy, which seemed so unfair. Frustrating conversation followed with the baby's father, who wanted her to have an abortion, a choice incompatible with her religious convictions. Later came the inevitable disclosure to her parents and their crushing reminder of how, to them, she so often appeared irresponsible. Through it all, she struggled to take responsibility. She sensed that she was taking control of her own life as she found enthusiasm for the pregnancy and a basis for hope. She came to love the baby growing inside her and eagerly anticipated celebrating its birth and raising it at home, with her parents' considerably grudging support. Then, all was taken away from her in those terrible hours of labor that ended in stillbirth. She thought, "How can the world be so cruel?"

Alone in the recovery room she is in considerable physical pain, but mostly she is stunned by what has happened. Her hopes dashed, she wishes it were all a bad dream. In silence, she longs to see her baby smile, to touch and kiss it, to feel its warmth in her arms and at her breast, to rock it, play with it, and sing it to sleep. She wonders how she can love her baby if she can't even take it home. She believes no one capable of understanding what she is experiencing and doubts she ever will share her innermost feelings with anyone. In some moments she feels very childlike and resolves to continue to expect her baby. Seeing how unrealistic this is, she is mildly tempted to retreat to her parents' sheltering arms. However, she feels shamed by her parents and dreads their ever hinting that this ending "might be for the best." She is vaguely aware that this is a watershed experience in her life that will change her permanently. Having read a book about dying and grief, she anticipates enduring "stages" of grief and painful healing. She has no idea how she will survive this onslaught.

As Jennifer lies in the recovery room, her parents, John and Denise, contact Terry, a funeral director, and request a quick and simple cremation. They hope to protect Jennifer from additional pain and suffering. They act as they believe parents should and without her consent. Terry denies the request and refuses to proceed without Jennifer's informed agreement. He insists that he must first speak with her. To fail to do so, he asserts, would be malpractice. Although he acknowledges their well-meaning concern, he tells John and Denise that his first obligation is to their daughter. He explains that it is, after all, primarily her experience and adjustment that are at stake and her vulnerability that calls for his professional response. John and Denise, somewhat hesitantly, grant Terry's request to meet with Jennifer.

Terry introduces himself to Jennifer, tells her what her parents have proposed and explains why he thinks it important to talk to her first. It is her experience, he says, and he wants to know what her wishes are. He says he can do as her parents ask, provided he knows that it is what she really wants. He tells her of decisions to be made before he can proceed but insists that she take time to think and not give her answers until he returns the next day. Among the decisions:

1) Does she want a funeral or immediate cremation? 2) Does she want her parents to pay? 3) If there is a funeral, does she want to attend? He can delay the service until she leaves the hospital or arrange for it to be held there. 4) Does she want to see her baby? 5) Does she want to name it? 6) Does she want the father to know, and does she want the father's name entered on the death certificate? 7) How, if at all, does she want to select a casket? 8) Does she want a minister? The session taxes Jennifer, but she feels no pressure for decisions on the spot. She cries but appreciates being asked. She thanks Terry for his sensitivity. She is relieved to have time to think about what she wants to do.

Terry returns the next day. Jennifer wants to see the baby later at the funeral home. She wants to attend a funeral and burial. She selects a modest casket sight unseen. She insists on paying for the funeral herself, although her resources are limited. She will make minimal payments over time. She will name the baby Bryan Timothy. And, she will ask the father for permission to put his name on the death certificate. This surprises Jennifer, since when first asked she had not wanted even to tell him of the birth because of his preference for abortion. (Later, he gives the permission.) At their first meeting she had told Terry of a bad experience with a priest and said, "There will be no priests. I hate them." In response, Terry told her of a gentle priest he knew. After a day's reflection, she says she is interested. (The priest is contacted later, and Jennifer finds comfort in his words and as they pray.)

Before leaving, Terry explains how he will wrap the baby in receiving blankets and place him in the casket. She can bring anyone she wants to the funeral home. Terry will show her the room where Bryan is to be laid in a closed casket. She will be able to choose how she wants to experience it. If she changes her mind, that will be fine.

On the day of the funeral, Jennifer comes to the funeral home alone an hour and a half before the service. Terry shows her where Bryan is and asks if she prefers going in alone or with him. She enters the room alone and closes the door behind her. Over an hour later she emerges with a reddened face. Prior to the service, Terry reenters the room and opens the casket. Pinned to the now rearranged receiving blankets is a note that says simply, "God will care for you."

After the funeral and the burial, Jennifer faces many challenges as she seeks to make a life for herself. She returns to a home where a nursery awaits a baby who is not coming. Her parents unsettle her, and she seeks a new peace with them. Relations with friends are strained. They seem so immature. She resents especially those who dismiss her loss and say such things as "Thank God you didn't know the baby" or "You're young; you can have another." She knows she must deal with this loss before ever thinking of another baby. She doubts her ability to bear children and her capacities to raise them. The pregnancy sidetracked her college plans, and she wonders if she can manage payments to the local junior college without help from her parents. She is uncertain about long-term goals and her capacities to "do anything right." She wonders if it is reasonable to be hopeful in a world where so much seems out of control. She feels good about her experience at the time of the funeral, and her memories of it and Terry's kindness support her fragile optimism.

Bereavement Is Choiceless, But Grieving Is Not

When Myra and Bryan die, Martin and Louise, and Jennifer feel helpless. Myra's languishing prior to death leaves Martin relieved when her suffering ends. The unrelenting sequence of events seems to him brutally unfair, and the bleak prospects for Fred reinforce his feelings of helplessness. He also fears that the children will begin to suspect that lack of choice threatens to make life intolerable. Louise's helplessness is so powerful that she seems to prefer refusing to accept the choiceless event of her mother's death to facing the reality of it. Jennifer is deeply troubled by the seeming unfairness and arbitrariness, first of her pregnancy and later of Bryan's death. Her ability to trust the world's safety is shaken; so much seems beyond her control.

It is vital that we reject ideas of grieving as passive and embrace ideas of it as active. By definition, bereavement *happens to* us. Indeed, *bereave* means "to deprive, to dispossess or strip from." Losing someone close through death is among our most wrenching experiences. Several years ago a woman in one of my workshops called death and bereavement "choiceless events." Since then, I have found no better way to express the helplessness of bereavement. As survivors, we control little of death's timing or character. Most of us, with a choice, would will that the dead live. Even when we welcome death as an inevitable end to suffering, we would avoid the suffering or the inevitability if we could. Many of us experience loss and its impacts as thrust on us by external forces. The lack of choice makes us feel that the world is out of control and that we are powerless to influence major events in our lives. Heightened anxiety, depression, and immobilization often ensue, and some of us slip into passivity and prolonged helplessness.

Much current writing suggests that grieving, too, is choiceless. We are told that grieving is yet another something that happens to us when we are bereaved, a process into which we are thrust against our will, that we must somehow survive. Bereavement is awful in part for these reasons, and when grieving is thought of in this way, we often dread it as more of the same. Like so many of us, Martin, Louise, and Jennifer are apprehensive about their own grieving, and what they've heard and read reinforces their apprehension. Such aversion to grieving dangerously inhibits us from actively coming to terms with what happens to us.

Grief Is an Emotion, Grieving a Coping Process

The specific emotion, grief, differs from the coping process, grieving. Grief holds a prominent place in our lives as survivors, but it is only a part of what we experience and do. As one of the most important impacts of bereavement, it is no part of our coping, although it may have a role in preparing us for grieving. The emotion comes over us and, in its extreme form, threatens to preoccupy us. Grieving as coping requires that we respond actively, invest energy, and address tasks. Among other things, coping requires that we come to terms with our grief emotion.

Grief, Motivation, and Helplessness

Martin, Louise, and Jennifer have established life patterns built around the expected presence of Myra and Bryan. Much of Martin's and Louise's daily routines that revolved around caring for Myra are no longer viable, although their emotional, behavioral, intellectual, and spiritual dispositions remain. Martin feels pangs of the emotion grief when his new reality regularly reminds him that his old dispositions no longer make sense. He feels love and affection for Myra but cannot express or show them in the usual ways. He catches himself about to call her, on the way to impossible visits, or using her name as if she were still alive. Louise, far more than Martin, continues to act on her old dispositions as she, for example, still brings food and clippings to the home to give to Mrya. Her strong reaction to the voice on the other end of the phone that tells her Myra is no longer at the home suggests she is determined to persist as if Myra lives. She thinks of Myra's suffering and hopes that it will end soon when it already has. Jennifer feels the emotion grief when she longs to hold her living newborn in the hospital, feels her love for

Bryan but cannot express or show it to him, realizes that she cannot take him home to the nursery she prepared for him, and sees that her plans, hopes and dreams for him are dashed.

The emotion grief is a complex experience, combining elements of belief, disposition, and pain and anguish. When we experience this emotion we believe that we have lost. Yet, we are disposed to feel, act, think, expect, and hope as if we have not lost. That is, we do not abruptly adopt a new posture in the world but rather remain postured as we were before the death. We are still disposed to care about and live with the one who has died. The emotion comes when we feel pain and anguish (sometimes visceral) over the impossibility of living out these dispositions. How can we possibly care about and for them if they are gone? How can we possibly not care for them?

When Martin and Jennifer are caught up short by reality and find themselves wanting reality to be different as their dispositions persist, they are not irrational. As they long for Myra and Bryan, they are all too painfully aware of the impossibility of their return. And they feel this pain exquisitely. For a time, they would just as soon not think about changing. They pull back from their harsh new realities and dwell for a time in their longing where they hold to the familiar dispositions to care about Myra and Bryan as if they were still present. What's the rush in coping? At first, they long intensely. But gradually they begin to face the challenges of putting together lives without Myra and Bryan, and their longing becomes less intense and constant.

We are not irrational when we entertain wishes or think contrary to fact. When we grieve, we commonly wish that the deceased were still alive. We feel the pain and anguish of grief as we realize in every corner of our worlds that they are no longer present. We must invest time and effort to change our daily lives and the dispositions that have served us well when those we cared about were with us. We are not irrational when we recoil from an all too painful new reality in order to muster the resources to cope with it. In the recoil (a temporary retreat from reality that must be faced eventually), our longing for those we cared about and the life pattern in which they held central places is not irrational. Our longing ordinarily remains wishful and nostalgic, albeit painful. Like Martin and Jennifer, and like most bereaved people, we recoil only temporarily. Our longing gradually becomes more episodic and intermittent as we turn our attention to finding new ways of living without those who died.

Louise appears to be heading toward a far more extreme grief as her desire for her mother's return intensifies. She seems intent on going on as if Myra has not died. She persists in familiar dispositions and behaviors, for example calling the home to speak to Myra or cutting the newspaper clippings and bringing them to her there. As she does so, she holds to familiar, though no longer viable, ways of expressing love for her mother. Her longing does not subside but rather deepens and preoccupies her. She seems determined to refuse to acknowledge the major change Myra's death entails and the challenges it presents. She is not merely pulling back from her new reality to catch her breath. Rather, she seems to be turning her back on the reality. She is clearly not eager or ready to change her life pattern by meeting new challenges. The longer she searches for Myra and fails to find her, the more likely her frustration and helplessness will mount.

When mourners go on as if a temporary retreat from reality is a sustainable posture in the world, they do something far different from temporarily indulging a wish that the world were other than it is. Grief leads some mourners to long for the return of the deceased in a way that if it persists, becomes irrational and dangerous. When they enter what I call extreme grief emotion, their disposition to expect, and their quite rational wish for, the presence of the deceased becomes a fervent, pervasive, preoccupying, and irrational desire. As they wholeheartedly and persistently desire the impossible and dwell in intense longing for what is irretrievably lost and recognized by them to be so, they experience something far different from ordinary grief. They are irrational precisely because their disposition to relate to the deceased as if he or she still lives flies in the face of their recognition, however painful, of her death. Their desire cannot be satisfied because their belief that the death has taken place is based on fact. In their intense longing, those who fall into extreme grief fervently want the impossible while they remain aware of its impossibility. The tension is not long sustainable and can lead, as it appears to be doing in Louise's case, to a suppression of the belief and a consequent refusal to face and to come to terms with death's reality.

Not only is extreme grief emotion irrational; it is dangerous. Generally, our emotions motivate us. They give us reasons to act. Think of when we are afraid, angry, in love or full of hate, for example. Our ordinary grief is the pain we feel when we are inappropriately disposed and postured in the face of a harsh new reality. In some cases (including Martin's and Jennifer's), ordinary grief leads us to desire to alter those dispositions to feel, act, think, expect, and hope that are not longer viable. Then ordinary grief motivates us to shape new life patterns appropriate to our new realities. That is, it motivates us to cope, to act constructively in response to what has happened to us. In particular, ordinary grief can lead us to desire to find new ways of loving the deceased in their absence. By contrast, for mourners like Louise, ordinary grief leads to extreme grief and the fervent desire for the return of the deceased. Mourners then become resolved to hold to dispositions to feel, act, think, expect and hope that are no longer viable—that is, to continue on as if the deceased still lived. In particular, extreme grief leads some of us (like Louise) to desire the return of the deceased and to continue in no longer viable ways of loving them. Herein lies the danger of extreme grief. The fervent desire for the return of the deceased that is at the core of extreme grief motivates no action, for there simply are no means to the end desired. Only denial can be motivated here. The belief that the deceased has died and the desire that this irreplaceable other be restored are incompatible, yet sustained together. As the desire and therefore the grief emotion intensify, those caught in extreme grief become frustrated, immobilized, helpless, and potentially paralyzed. The depth and power of extreme grief derive from this lack of motivational force. The pain and anguish of extreme grief become excruciating just because there is nothing those caught in it can say or do to bring back those they care about. Extreme grief emotion provides no ground for hope, only ground for despair.

It is misleading and dangerous for us to mistake the emotion grief for the whole of bereavement—misleading because our experience encompasses diverse physical, psychological/emotional, behavioral, social, and intellectual/spiritual effects in our shattered lives and dangerous because precisely this aspect of bereavement potentially debilitates us most when we take it to its extreme. Sustained focus on extreme grief can easily incline us to think that grieving is passive, disease-like, and debilitating. Frustrated helplessness in yearning for the impossible return of the deceased compounds difficulties for some who do not know how to go on with their lives. When mourners experience extreme grief emotion, it interferes as they address other challenges.

The Attractions of Grief

Dwelling in the emotion grief attracts and captivates some mourners. Paradoxically, although they want control, they sometimes remain (seemingly willfully) in the extreme grief where they can find no control. Why does this happen?

Martin feels abandoned by his elderly mother. Though he had long since established a life and family on his own, still he feels the tug of attachment to her. Jennifer grew attached to Bryan in her womb, then experienced the pain of the rupture of the bonds at the moment of birth. Martin and Jennifer's losses arouse grief and longing in them as the biological child and parent they are. Their yearning is an organic impact of Myra's and Bryan's deaths. Martin and Jennifer, however, soon begin once again to face reality and to pick up the pieces of their shattered lives. Louise too feels abandoned by her mother, though she appears to feel it more acutely. Her longing intensifies. Her behaviors become inappropriate to her new reality as she goes on as if Myra were still alive. She does not turn to face her new reality but lingers in retreat from it.

There is no doubt there is something biological about ordinary grief emotion that has to do with *deeply ingrained attachment patterns in our lives*. John Bowlby[1] emphasizes the inportance of bonding at a preconscious, biological level. Attachment is vital for the survival and flourishing of the social vertebrates, especially the higher primate and human species. On this view, when we mourn, our retreat from activity in grief is an organic, evolutionarily reinforced, protective defense mechanism employed in the face of something we perceive as threatening. It is an instance of the well-known flight or fight response. As we reel in response to the hurt of the loss itself and to the threats it represents, we withdraw in grief to guard against further hurt and to brace organically to meet whatever challenges might come next. Ordinarily, this works temporarily, and we begin to cope actively when we are ready. For some of us, like Louise, however, the reeling continues; they are rendered unable to deal with reality by their sustained numbing and their withdrawal in extreme grief. Their behaviors become rigid and ritualistic. As they yearn and search for the deceased, they persist automatically in behaviors that once either held the deceased near or brought them back from previous separations. They remain bonded biologically in ways they little recognize.

Martin recognizes the challenges in Fred's increasing dependence and in reconstructing his own family life. He is daunted by them. He pauses, as the bereaved commonly do. Jennifer senses that her experience is a major turning point in her young life. She hesitates to define the new shape of her life. In contrast, Louise's retreat from reality endures. In it she neither acknowledges nor addresses the challenges her new reality presents.

Some of us may retreat into ordinary grief as *a semideliberate, and perhaps psychologically necessary, hesitation* before we actively cope with loss. This psychological retreat from effort may serve us well temporarily, but when we remain in retreat, it does not. However dimly or fully we understand the challenges before us, we normally recognize that our losses require that we make major changes in our lives. When we linger in grief and retreat futher from reality, we resist or delay such change and transformation; we accept the comforts of passivity rather than exert the considerable effort required to come to terms with so much all at once.

Martin knows well a world with Myra's companionship for Fred and Myra's illness as a ready and legitimate excuse for relative neglect of his own family. The new landscape carved by Myra's death is strange and forbidding. Yet he faces it. Jennifer has held Bryan as a central focus in her life for months. The prospect of moving out from under her parents' sometimes excessive protection seems more than she knows how to handle. Still, she is intent on doing so. Louise, by contrast, unconsciously seeks to avoid dealing with her new and radically different life circumstances in her persistent longing for Myra's return and as she struggles to sustain a no longer viable, but still comfortable and familiar, life pattern.

When we mourn, we confront the unkown of life without those we have cared about. Some of us, like Louise, may *stay in grief to avoid the unknown.* We know life where desire for the now dead is prominent. As we keep the desire alive, we still want the security that the desire brought before the death. The known is relatively safe. If we allow the desire for the deceased to extinguish, we risk living where the security is no longer available.

Phillip, a well-to-do, childless widower in his forties, has allowed his life to remain in disarray long after his wife Adrienne's death. The outpouring of concern for him and of love for his wife at her funeral was deeply moving and gratifying, and he has remained dependent on others ever since. Whenever anyone mentions Adrienne, he sobs openly and appears overwhelmed. This elicits sympathy and comfort from family and friends alike. Phillip had depended on Adrienne for his social life and rarely took any initiative. Now he depends on other survivors and is never disappointed. His and Adrienne's parents see how he still misses her terribly, and they go out of their way to console him and make sure he is not home alone in the evenings. Friends see how lost he is without her and regularly invite him out. Feeling sorry for him, they include him just as he would have been included had his wife lived. Phillip's private consulting practice has fallen off markedly, but he was about to retire early anyway and does not need the money. His associates express sympathy for how hard it must be to care about other people's affairs, and they deal with him very forgivingly. He talks of his wife as the center of the life they knew with others. He says, "I don't think anyone would be paying attention to me had Adrienne not been so wonderful. I don't know what would happen to me if the others sensed I was over losing her." For Phillip, the comforts of remaining in grief are many. He has little incentive to take initiative and put together a new, independent life.

For people like Phillip, *remaining in grief brings secondary rewards*. Family, friends, and associates see their protracted longing, yearning, and searching, and these outward signs of grief bring at least attention and often sympathy, understanding, patience, and efforts to comfort and support that the bereaved find gratifying. Some who, like Phillip, linger in grief may fear that as they move beyond grief, others will withdraw the attention, comfort, and support they crave. If any of them perceive themselves as truly helpless, as Phillip may, the felt need for secondary rewards may intensify. Some of us semiconsciously or unwittingly adopt a posture of permanent grieving in order to hold on to these secondary rewards.

Martin and Louise are at a loss as to how to hear and speak words unspoken with Myra. They long to know that she loved them despite the decision to place her and Fred in the nursing home. They wish she were present so that they could hear her words of forgiveness and so that they could reconcile. They wish they could show her how much they still love her. Martin may soon be ready to learn how to love Myra in her absence. In contrast, Louise seems convinced that Myra's presence is utterly necessary. She fears that she cannot go on without Myra, and her desire for her return nearly preoccupies her. Jennifer wonders, as she lies alone in the recovery room, how she can love Bryan if she cannot take him home until Terry helps her begin to express her love in Bryan's absence.

We do not stop loving or caring about those who die when they die. In fact, most mourners I have known fervently resist any suggestion that they must, or eventually will, do so. One of the most important aspects of grieving is finding ways to make a transition from caring about others who are present to caring about them when they are absent.[2] Some of us may remain in grief for *fear that if they stop longing for those they have lost, they will stop loving them.*

This they fervently do not want to do. They desire to be with the deceased, as the desire to be together was central to the pattern of loving prior to the death. If they know no other way to sustain the love, they may hold onto that desire even though it frustrates them. Like Louise, they may be able to relinquish the desire for the impossible only when they find alternative means of sustaining their love.

A teen-aged young man, Rick, whose mother died unexpectedly, stills lives at home with his father. It has been over a year since his mother's death, and yet Rick insists that his father and siblings leave utterly nothing changed at home. Virtually everything she left behind, including her clothing and even her toothbrush, remain just where they were when she died. And he insists that the family's daily routine remain what it was, including setting an empty place at the table. He maintains this degree of control by threatening angry outbursts aimed at any who take exception. Rick said to me with his chin thrust forward, "I don't see why anything has to change." He clearly resists dealing with the unknown world where a change that makes a major difference in his and his family's life has already taken place. Rick's world is now radically different, but he refuses to face it. Every day, and in virtually every corner of his home, he both sees that his mother is not there and insists on holding on to a pattern of living that carries on as if she were.

Paradoxically, in their grief some mourners *refuse to accept the loss as real in the face of that very reality*. This refusal may be imbedded in a more encompassing refusal to acknowledge and accept limitation, vulnerability, and powerlessness. In grief some of us, like Rick, may blindly defy the human condition with our eyes open. Such defiance may be for a time psychologically or emotionally necessary when no other hopeful exertions of the will appear available. Some of us may find it pointless to pursue any other desires or to try to shape a new life unless and until something at least nearly as desirable as life with the deceased comes into view. In this, as perhaps in all suffering, there is a profound inertia and, in some instances, a stubbornness or perseverance that immobilizes those who suffer. Martin hates the seemingly unfair and unrelentingly cruel reality, but his abiding feelings of responsibility for Fred and especially for his own family motivate him to cope actively. Louise, by contrast, appears to be refusing to accept her new reality and unable to see the point of shaping a new life. Jennifer is tempted to refuse to accept the reality of her loss; she wishes it were all a bad dream. Terry's interventions support her as she resists this temptation.

We Must Choose to Overcome Grief

Several of these motivations pull each of us to dwell in grief. The danger is that we will become mired in extreme grief unless others encourage and support us as we cope with the challenges we face. Extreme grief prevents some of us from acting to meet those challenges, from actively grieving. This danger lends a kernel of truth to the medical view of grief that stresses the need for detachment from the deceased. Although successful coping does not require that we completely let go, it does require that we let go of the irrational desire for the impossible that is embedded in extreme grief. We must dissipate the debilitating and potentially paralyzing extreme emotion and shift our focus to coping actively.

When we are bereaved, we need motivation to break from the emotion grief in order to get on with grieving as coping. Ordinarily the dissonance between our no longer viable dispositions and our new reality motivates us to modify those dispositions and the life patterns they drive. Whatever attracts and holds any one of us in the emotion grief, the first step in coping is to resist its attractions, to break its hold. As we resist, we no longer perceive ourselves as helpless victims of choiceless death events. Instead, we adopt a new active posture as persons who can do and say at least something meaningful in the face of our losses. We no longer passively absorb the disarray in our lives and resolve to come to terms with it. We do not simply look forward to enduring more choiceless experience after death. We can take some small beginning steps to accept and take on challenges and shape new life patterns and the next chapters of our lives.

We should not underestimate the difficulty of moving beyond grief. The pain of the shattering of our lives is considerable. We find comfort as we numb ourselves and retreat from dealing with the harsh new reality and the chaos in our lives. We may need temporary retreat. Physical, psychological, behavioral, social, and spiritual inertia inhibit our progress. Some mourners become physically exhausted and lose all energy for living. Some feel anxious, frightened, helpless, or powerless. Some are reluctant to change deeply engrained desires, motivations, dispositions, and habits; some are simply stubborn. Still others hesitate to seek or accept support from anyone. Some mourners feel hopeless and find it hard to acknowledge or accept their own limits and vulnerability. Together, these influences conspire against moving on. Still, the choice to struggle against the attractions of the emotion grief is the first, and surely among the most fundamental, choice(s) mourners must make if they are to begin coping. In effect, when we are bereaved we choose whether to remain in deprivation, immersed in the impacts of bereavement, or to start coming to terms with that deprivation and move on to new experience and a new pattern of life despite our losses.

Some Say We Grieve in Stages or Phases

Writers and speakers on grieving commonly tell us that as we grieve we go through stages or phases that enter our lives one after another. In social scientific and clinical writing, Erich Lindemann tells us that we grieve in three stages: shock and disbelief, acute mourning, and resolution.[3] John Bowlby says we grieve in three phases: the urge to recover the lost object, disorganization and despair, and reorganization.[4] George Engel's six-stage idea includes shock and disbelief, development of awareness, restitution, resolution of the loss, idealization, and outcome.[5] Colin Murray Parkes modified Bowlby's idea (and Bowlby later accepted the modification) to describe four phases of grieving: numbness, yearning and searching, disorganization and despair, and reorganization.[6] Popular writings are dominated by the view of Elisabeth Kubler-Ross that we grieve in five stages: shock and denial, anger, bargaining, depression, and acceptance.[7] The list of such ideas could be extended indefinitely; commonly accessible writings on grieving contain an abundance of such ideas. Martin and Louise heard a similar account in the nursing home talk, and Jennifer read it in her book. More often than not, when I talk to mourners, they readily recite some such account of what they are supposedly experiencing or are about to experience.

Without engaging in a detailed review of these ideas, I ask that you note the common pattern they contain: We are told that when we grieve, we are first hit hard by our bereavement. We are then immersed in the full impact of intense and often nearly overwhelmingly painful experiences. Eventually, however, we achieve some kind of new equilibrium in living as if we had been washed up on shore after having nearly drowned. To elaborate more fully: When we grieve, we first experience such things as shock, disbelief, longing, preoccupation with the deceased and an acute awareness of sights, sounds, or smells that call the person to mind, yearning and searching for the deceased, numbness, withdrawal in defense, and denial. After this initial phase, we are thrown into the middle phase in which we experience the full force of bereavement as manifested by somatic distress, symptoms like those experienced by the deceased, restlessness, and irritability. We are burdened with acute and intense emotions such as sadness, depression, anxiety, despair, helplessness, anger, frustration, and guilt. Some of us cling to idealizations of the deceased. We are said to lose motivation for daily life and experience the breakdown of familiar behavior patterns. We become isolated from others, and some of us fail in negotiation with others (including God) to change the unacceptable new reality. We fall into purposelessness and hopelessness. In the final stage, we experience such things as subsiding somatic effects and reduction in the intensity of our emotion and preoccupation with the deceased. Our emotional equilibrium is restored, and we come to accept what has happened. We reestablish social contacts and adopt new roles and skills. We remember those who have died without pain and loosen ties to them. We are restored to daily purpose and hopefulness.

Many writers caution that we do not automatically flow through the stages or phases, and suggest that the phases overlap as we experience them. Many observers assert that we do not fall into lockstep as we grieve or lose our individuality. All, however, emphasize the physical, emotional, behavioral, social, and intellectual consequences that we endure in some predictable sequence.

Some Describe Our Grieving in Medical Terms

Some writers and speakers tell us that when we are bereaved, it is as if we have had an illness thrust on us of suffered a wound. They continue these medical analogies as they tell us that our grieving is like healing or recovery. Lindemann describes the "symptomatology and management" of acute grief and likens grieving to a psychiatric illness.[8] Engel suggests that grief is like a disease with a classic syndrome of symptoms and likens grieving to a healing process.[9] Parkes says that grief is a functional psychiatric disorder of known etiology, with distinctive features and a relatively predictable course. But he prefers to draw an analogy between grieving and recovery from a physical injury or wound.[10]

Once again, without examining these accounts in detail, I ask that you note the common pattern: Each writer tells us that as we grieve, we manifest so-called "symptoms" of grieving, including somatic distress (tight throat, shortness of breath, sighing, emptiness in the abdomen, lack of muscular power, and tension), crying, and numbing. We become helpless, attempt to resist taking in the reality of the death, become preoccupied with the deceased (often attaching ourselves to a mental image of the deceased), or become identified with traits of the deceased. We feel guilt and anger, and we often fall into hopelessness and despair. We react with hostility, and our usual patterns of behavior break down. We incur troubles in personal interactions. Each of these writers tell us that our grieving is a healing process. Parkes writes that, as with healing from wounds, our grieving may result either in healing, healing with complications (including scars), failure to heal, or reopening.

Writers and speakers continue to debate whether talking of grieving in such medical terms is appropriate. I have attended many conferences where I have seen and heard lively exchanges among clinicians and professionals. Therese Rando details many ways in which she believes that "complicated" grieving cries for clinical attention.[11] Beverly Raphael urges that although pathological complications in grieving may be more readily equated with illness, the medical analogy is more difficult to sustain with uncomplicated grief.[12] Other writers adamantly protest that grieving, as a normal process of adaptation to loss, is not analogous to disease, no matter its course.[13] As the professional debate continues, popular writings and common understanding still refer to "symptoms" of grieving and grieving as healing or recovery.

Is It Helpful to Talk of Stages, Phases, and Medical Analogies?

Neither the idea that grieving is something that unfolds in stages or phases, nor the idea that it is like recovering or healing from an illness or wound provides what mourners or those who care about them seek. For one thing, *the ideas do not provide an adequate general understanding.* Advocates of both ideas blur the distinction between what happens to us when we are bereaved and what we do as we grieve in response. They emphasize how our experiences unfold passively in expectable sequences or liken our grieving to our manifesting symptoms of disease or passively healing from a wound.[14] As they do so, they treat coping as something that happens to us when we lose. "Give it time," they so often tell us, but they say little about the effort our coping requires. They miss how essentially active we are when we grieve. None discusses the varieties of challenge we face or stresses the crucial role of choice in our responses to choiceless events.

Proponents of the medical analogy also suggest erroneously

(and perhaps unwittingly) in their talk of symptoms, illness, and injury that there is something wrong with or abnormal about us when we grieve. Although this suggestion may be appropriate as they describe pathological or complicated bereavement, it doesn't ring true with many of us as we experience our grieving as the quite normal thing to do when someone dies.

Proponents of the medical analogy tend to focus on specific facets of grieving and miss how we grieve as whole persons, in all facets of our being. They often talk as if we respond somatically, emotionally or psychologically, behaviorally, socially, or intellectually or spiritually in splendid isolation. Some focus exclusively, or nearly exclusively, on one facet of our grieving in a way that mistakes that facet for the whole.

Finally, both ideas wrongly suggest that we come to an end in our grieving as we either complete the stages or at last recover. In effect, they suggest that we can somehow finish coping with mystery. Although when we grieve we often can and do return to settled living patterns, as these ideas tell us, the mysteries that prompt us to renewed grieving can always unsettle us and our ways of living.

In each of these ways, the ideas of stages of grieving and the use of medical analogies either fail to resonate with our experiences when we are bereaved and grieve or actually distort our self-understanding. In turn, they distort the understanding of others who wish to support or comfort us. Broadly accessible as the ideas may be, their very accessibility is no virtue when the ideas fail to capture the general shape and contour of our experiences of bereavement and of our coping responses.

Moreover, *these ideas do not give us means to respect individuality*. They emphasize how alike we are and how predictable as we grieve. In reality, however, we grieve neither so uniformly nor so predictably. Most such ideas take root in empirical studies of large populations of grieving persons. They are at best statistical generalizations describing what is probable across a particular population. But statements of probability say nothing specific about particular individuals. To see the point, consider that despite the statistical statement that the average couple has 2.1 children, no couple in fact has fractional children. None of us is a statistical or average person. We are flesh-and-blood individuals whose experiences vary considerably from any general tendencies captured in statements of probability. We live and grieve in those variations. The stage and phase and medical ideas of grieving provide no clues about the ranges of such variations in our living and grieving that others must come to know and appreciate if they are to respect the uniqueness of our experiences.

In addition, *the ideas may actually reinforce our feelings of helplessness* when we are bereaved. First death assaults us, we are told, and then our grieving carries us along inevitably through more choiceless events and experiences. We are either subjected to sequences of stages or phases or afflicted with a syndrome of symptoms. Given an indefinite amount of time and endurance, we eventually find ourselves at a stage or phase of reorientation or reorganization, or we are healed or recovered. On both views, we remain mostly passive and helpless, as we were when we faced the losses themselves. In other words, proponents seem to be telling us that after bereavement happens to us, grieving is something more that happens to us. Neither view tells us how long we may have to endure more of this passivity. Neither view stresses that when we grieve, we actively respond to what has happened to us. Neither view speaks of our having choice or control in our grieving. Much less does either give us any idea of the varieties of choices before us. I can think of no better way to reinforce our already troubling feelings of powerlessness and helplessness.

Finally, *both ideas provide little guidance for caregivers.* Most benignly, those who write and speak of stages or phases or in medical terms urge that caregivers wait with us, as the stages, phases, or healing run their course. They seem to be saying that, eventually, "this, too, will pass," as if grieving were a fog that finally lifts. In effect, proponents of the ideas urge caregivers to join us in our passivity. They encourage them to listen actively to, and comfort, us. They urge them to reassure us that what we passively endure is normal when it is. Neither idea offers any guidance for helping us as we actively respond to what has happened to us. Neither suggests ways of supporting us as we choose new daily life patterns or redirect our life stories.

More insidious, all too commonly, and despite the protests of some proponents of the ideas, caregivers often misuse the ideas to prescribe how we ought to grieve. As they do so, they suggest that there is a "proper" or "best" way for us to grieve. This bypasses and neglects our individuality and the uniqueness of our life circumstances and experiences.

Many scholarly and popular writers who use these models define helping as doing for the bereaved who cannot do for themselves. For example, the repeated use of the expression "symptom management" suggests that much of our grieving is fostered by the efforts of others. They forget that only we can pick up the pieces of our shattered lives and move into their next chapters.

Some Say That as We Grieve, We Address Tasks

In contrast to both stage/phase and medical ideas about grieving, some writers stress the challenges that we face when we are bereaved and the tasks we must address in grieving. Lindemann was the first writer to use the expression "grief work" to characterize our grieving.[15] He identifies three principal tasks: relinquishing attachment to the deceased, adjusting to the environment where the deceased is missing, and developing new relationships. Parkes and Weiss identify three tasks: acknowledging and explaining our losses, emotionally accepting the losses, and assuming a new identity.[16] And William Worden outlines four tasks: acknowledging the reality of our losses, working through the emotional turmoil in our lives, adjusting to the environment where the deceased is absent, and loosening our ties to the deceased.[17]

Again, I will not go into the details of these accounts. I ask only that you note the similarities. On all accounts, our grieving is thought of as something that we do. We do not remain passive but rather actively engage the challenges presented by our longing for, and need to let go of, those we care about. We struggle to find means of overcoming, gaining control of, or constructively expressing and directing our emotions. We work our way through crises in self-identity and disruptions in our usual behavior patterns and develop alternatives. We address and seek to overcome strains in relationships and to build new ones. And we seek ways to make sense of our new reality and to find meaning in life without the deceased.

A Task-Based, Active View

William Worden tells us that when we are bereaved, we must complete the four tasks of grieving:

- *Acknowledge the reality of the loss.* We must overcome the temptation to deny or avoid the reality of our loss, fully acknowledge it, and recognize its implications for our life patterns.
- *Work through the emotional turmoil.* We must find effective means to work through and to express the emotions we

experience in the aftermath of loss, rather than avoid, circumvent or repress them.

- *Adjust to the environment where the deceased is absent.* We must define new life patterns that adjust appropriately and meaningfully for the fact that the deceased is missing.
- *Loosen ties to the deceased.* We must free ourselves from our bonds to the deceased in order once again to become involved with other persons. We must find effective means to say good-bye.[18]

I agree with Worden on several major points. It is best for us to focus on the grief work we must do in order to progress and to accommodate loss in our lives. We must do grief work in each of the areas he identifies. And we can best understand that grief work in terms of specific tasks that we must address. However, I believe that Worden's view needs refinement if it is to provide what persons seek in ideas about grieving as I have outlined them in Chapter 1; only a refined view can provide us with a useful and accessible general understanding, support respect for our individuality, support us in dealing with our helplessness, and provide useful guidance for our caregivers.

Worden mischaracterizes the items on his list as tasks. They simply are not tasks at all. Tasks, as I understand them and as dictionaries define them, are circumscribable, modest in scale, and completable. This is not true for any of the items he lists. Rather than identifying tasks, he identifies important facets of active coping. His four "tasks" correspond nicely to the four principal facets of coping that I identify in Chapter 1. His "acknowledging the reality of the loss" corresponds to the intellectual and spiritual facet of our coping in which we struggle to take in the reality of, and make sense of, our losses. His "working through the emotional turmoil" amounts to the emotional and psychological facet of our coping in which we acknowledge our feelings and express or otherwise process them. His "adjusting to the environment where the deceased in absent" corresponds to the behavioral facet of our coping as we explore and adopt the life pattern changes that our losses demand. And finally, his "loosening ties to the deceased" corresponds to the social facet of our coping as we find a new way to relate to those we have lost and accommodate the loss in relationships with our fellow survivors.[19] Moreover, to the extent that our making and changing social relationships has biological significance, the correspondence pattern also encompasses the biological facet of our coping. Of course, our coping in that dimension is organic, and we are not fully conscious of it.

As I said in Chapter 1, when we cope with loss, we cope as whole persons, involving all major facets of our being at once. I agree with Worden that our coping has all of these major facets. However, our coping is not tasklike in any of these major facets of our lives. When we mourn, like Martin, Louise, and Jennifer, we will continue to confront parts of reality and be challenged to acknowledge and make sense of the differences entailed by our losses until we die. So, too, throughout the remainder of our lives, wherever and whenever we are reminded of those we have lost, we will experience episodes of feeling and emotion, continue to adapt to our changed environments, and renegotiate relationships with the dead and with our fellow survivors. To put it another way, we will cope intellectually and spirtually, emotionally and psychologically, behaviorally, socially, and biologically with the major losses in our lives as long as we live. The items on Worden's list are thus not tasks, rigorously defined; they are not circumscribable, modest in scale, or completable.

By contrast with Worden's view, the idea that I develop and elaborate in later chapters is that the combination of tasks that we confront when we are bereaved requires that we relearn the world. The types of tasks we must address include coming to terms with the physical world of things, places, and events and our "spiritual place" in the world; the social world of others, including our fellow survivors, the dead, and, in some cases, God; and aspects of our selves at the centers of our unique experiences of the world. Clearly, coming to terms with the physical world, the social world, and ourselves is no more circumscribable, modest in scale, or completable than are the items Worden lists. Coping with particular aspects of these undertakings, however, amounts to addressing tasks properly so called. We can identify a particular challenge we wish to address, decide what to do for the time being, take action on the matter, and then move on to other things. Typical tasks of this sort include, for examples, coming to terms with a particular thing or place (a picture of Myra, an item of clothing bought for Bryan, or a place at our kitchen table); having a specific conversation (Martin or Louise with Fred or a nurse at the home, Jennifer with either parent, or any of us with our closest friend); or deciding when to return to work (Martin), finding more time to be a mother to one's youngest child (Louise), declaring one's independence by finding a place of one's own (Jennifer), or deciding to return to an activity that the one who died introduced into one's life.

As we address tasks of these types, we engage the challenges they present as the whole persons we are, that is, in all of the facets Worden identifies simultaneously. Our coping with loss in all facets of our lives is of a piece. Each facet of our coping is intimately connected with every other facet.

Consider Martin as he addresses the task of coming to terms with the chair from Myra's home that she gave him when she entered the nursing home and that now sits in his family room. He can choose whether to discard or store it, avoid it, vow never to sit in it again, sit in it until he can't stand it, or sit in it to draw comfort from feeling close to his mother. As he makes his choice, he acknowledges and makes sense of a part of his reality transformed by the loss, that is, the chair and the fact that his mother will never be seated in it again. He feels and possibly expresses a wide range of emotion. As he enacts his decision, he begins to behave differently in a small corner of his world. He renegotiates his relationships with his mother and others.

As another example, consider Jennifer's conversation with Bryan's father in which she asks permission to put the father's name on the death certificate. She can choose whether to have the conversation at all, when she wants to talk with him, how she will approach him, and what she really wants from him. As she enacts her decision to talk with him, she acknowledges and makes sense of a part of her reality (her relationship with Bryan's father) that has been transformed by the loss. No doubt she feels emotion, and she may or may not express it in many ways. She behaves differently as she renegotiates her relationship with the father. She also takes responsibility for the last details of Bryan's life.

As one last example, consider a specific decision you have had to make about giving new direction to your life when someone has died, for example, whether to continue in an activity that the deceased had introduced into your life. You could have chosen, for example, to stop doing it for some period of time, or to continue to do it alone, or to ask someone else to join you. As you considered your options, you acknowledged and made sense of a part of your reality (you could no longer do this thing with the deceased). No doubt you felt and possibly expressed emotion as you chose and began to live with the choice. You found a new place for an old behavior in your life pattern or set aside the activity. As you did so, you were saying a good-bye to the one you loved and possibly joining someone else in a new way.

| | Worden's "Tasks" / Facets of Coping | | | |
	Acknowledge loss/ Intellectual/spiritual	Express emotion/ Psychological	Learn to live again/ Behavioral	Let go/ Social
Attig's Relearning the World Tasks				
Physical world				
Social world				
One's self				
The deceased				

This chart depicts the relationship between Worden's account and the one I develop in later chapters. The top arrays Worden's four "tasks" together with translations of them as facets of coping. The column on the left arrays the varieties of tasks that I believe together constitute the grief work of "relearning the world." The chart implies that for any task on the left, a mourner will be challenged to cope in all of the facets of his or her life as listed across the top. Because we cope as whole persons, our coping with any of the real tasks that make up grief work entails effort, and has consequences, in each facet of our lives.

We All Have Some Choices as We Grieve

Although many of us experience bereavement as a "choiceless" event, we have many choices in how we grieve. Consider some of the choices facing Martin, Louise, Jennifer, and any of us when we grieve. Although the ordinary grief emotion tends to invade our lives and spellbind us, we can indulge in it or we can struggle against what attracts us in it. This most basic choice requires a distinctive kind of hope, and optimism rooted in faith and conviction that supports and sustains the capacity to affirm life without the one we have loved and cared about. We, like Martin, Louise, and Jennifer, can pace ourselves, choose when to make our efforts, and adopt our own styles as we meet the challenges and address the tasks that the loss of the loved ones presents. We can attack the tasks and challenges vigorously and invest much time and energy in our grief work, or we can allow ourselves frequent respite from rigors of the process.

We, like Martin, Louise and Jennifer, can focus our attention where we will. We can interact with our loved one's body or refrain. We can encounter some of our physical surroundings and avoid others. We can witness or avoid events during the funeral period, such as casket closings or the burial. We can visit or stay away from places of significance. We can decide now or later whether to keep, discard, or set aside physical effects, pictures, mementos, and other significant objects.

We can express in our own ways, or keep to ourselves, the emotions we experience and the new meanings we discern. We can be spectators at the funeral or actively participate in such social responses to death, as Terry helps Jennifer to do. We can do or say what is meaningful to us either in private, as Jennifer does when alone with Bryan, or in the presence of others. We can withdraw from others' support, as Martin and Louise do, or reach out for or accept support or comfort, as Jennifer does to the priest and from Terry. We can respond to others' needs for support, as Martin does with Fred and his own children, or we can decline to help, perhaps until we feel better able to do so. We can decide how, if at all, to approach and interact with friends, relatives, and peers. We can build a new and dynamic relationship with the deceased, give shape to our lives in part through continuing, albeit transformed, interaction with the life now ended, as Martin longs to do and Jennifer begins to do in naming Bryan and commending him to God's care.

Like Martin, who hopes to spend less time at the nursing home and more with his family, and Jennifer, who determines to take more day-to-day responsibility for her actions, we can continue with all, part, or none of our daily routines. Like Martin, who wonders about the point of working, dreads, but does not abandon, his ongoing concern for Fred, and renews his commitment to his family, we can reassess, abandon, set aside temporarily, or return to our most important ongoing projects, activities, or commitments. Like Jennifer, who considers entering college, we can undertake new projects, activities, or commitments. We can hold fast to our most fundamental beliefs about what gives life and death meaning or search for new ways of standing before these mysteries.

This list of our choices is virtually endless. The examples I have given indicate that we face innumerable alternatives. Rather than being choiceless, bereavement is painfully challenging for us in part because we have so very many choices. Although some of our life before loss remains viable, so much of what we took for granted as settled is now unsettled, and we find it difficult to know how to begin to establish a new life pattern. Perhaps the emotion grief attracts us in this way: Longing for the deceased seems more settled to us than the unsettling alternative of facing an overwhelming array of choices.

I wish to be clear about my use of "choice" in this context, and about my meaning. As we respond to loss, our behaviors range along a continuum from strategic, highly self-reflective, and deliberate actions to minimally self-reflective, habitual, and semiautomatic behaviors. Unhappily, and I believe mistakenly, many of us think of choices only as outcomes of fully self-reflective deliberation. When we self-consciously examine and evaluate alternatives before we act, we choose in the fullest sense of the term. So it is that Martin and

Louise (albeit reluctantly) chose to move Myra and Fred to the nursing home. So, too, Jennifer accepted Terry's invitation to choose more self-reflectively among alternatives for Bryan's funeral. By this standard, choices would be rare in our lives.

We need not, however, deliberate so extensively before we choose. We can, and often do, choose and cope effectively and straightforwardly without such intense deliberation. We choose when alternatives are available to us, we are aware of them, and we are able to do otherwise. When we chose, our intentions produce our behaviors. We need not review and evaluate those intentions to choose; we need only act on them. However the intentions came to be ours, that is, part of our dispositional and motivational makeup or character, the actions and behaviors that result from them are truly ours and chosen by us. Martin feels frustrated when his ordinary ways of dealing with events in his life fail him after Myra dies. He feels a need to think more clearly about his alternatives. Only when, as for Martin, our usually effective, straightforward choosing and coping proves ineffective or frustrating may we feel a need to proceed more self-consciously and deliberatively.

We choose when we are free of the influence either of external forces beyond our control (for example, coercion by others or the effects of drugs). To choose, we must also be free of internal forces beyond our control (for example, compulsions, obsessions, or psychotic states). Despite the fact that bereavement brings great stress into our lives, it is implausible to presume that when we are bereaved we act compulsively or obsessively where we did not before. Only rarely do some people develop compulsions or obsessions in their bereavement. Of course, the stress we feel when we lose commonly makes more difficult, but not impossible, our efforts to see alternatives before us, weigh those alternatives (self-reflectively or however habitually we normally do so), or move ourselves to action. Martin and Jennifer experience all of these difficulties, but neither is compulsive or obsessive. Louise's intensifying longing for Myra's return verges on and could become both.

Grieving Is Active: A Summary

When we are bereaved, an event or series of events not of our choosing and well beyond our control has left our lives more or less in a shambles. Much has happened that cannot be undone, no matter how fervently we may desire it. Normally, we long for the return of those who have died and for the life we knew when they shared it with us. Although it makes no sense for us to continue in many of our desires, motivations, dispositions, behaviors, and habits in a reality transformed by our losses, we do so. It can seem that, no matter where we turn in our worlds, some thing, some place, or someone reminds us that we have lost. The world and our lives in it can never be as they were.

When the world reminds us of these things, we feel the pangs of grief. Some of us, like Phillip, Rick, and Louise, fall into extreme grief emotion where we linger, suspended before a new world we cannot or will not face. When we do so, we remain passive in a world that has already dealt us a severe blow. We risk prolonged helplessness and even paralysis as we do and say little to nothing to find a way of going on. If we are to pick up the pieces of our lives and go on without those who have died, we must resist whatever might attract us to lingering in grief. We must choose to cope rather than to succumb.

Coping requires that we actively respond to what has happened to us, that we change our daily life patterns and direction in life. We must meet challenges and address tasks as we come to terms with objects, places, and events; relationships with family members, friends, fellow survivors, the deceased, and, perhaps, God; and elements of our daily routines, work and leisure lives, ongoing projects and commitments, perhaps our fundamental beliefs, and our expectations and hopes for the future. We address these tasks as the whole persons we are. We all at once exert physical energy and bond biologically, work through and express emotion, change behavior, modify relationships, and make sense of our new reality and our new selves.

Although we have little to no choice in bereavement, choice pervades our grieving. As we address our tasks, we again and again choose among alternative steps into our futures. We do not, and cannot, cope with the whole world at once. There are always new landscapes to confront and new challenges to address. As we choose, new options open before us.

Reshaping our daily lives and changing course in our biographies are ongoing projects, never finally settled. Bereavement humbles us as it teaches us how easily what we have thought to be settled can be undone. So it is with any progress we make in grieving. We will never be "over" having lost those we have cared about, since the mysteries of life, death, and suffering remain untouched by our coping. We will have occasion to grieve our losses until we ourselves die.

The Idea Provides General Understanding

When I have shared this task-based idea of grieving as active with mourners, they have told me that it resonates at all points with their experiences. The idea orients them in the chaos bereavement introduces into their lives and to the variety of challenges and tasks they face every day, in every corner of their lives. They find self-understanding in this idea. They find reassurance that they are not alone in grieving, that others have faced similar challenges. And they find a general understanding that they wish were shared widely in the world around them, especially among those closest to them and those who seem to understand so little of what they are going through. The idea is broadly accessible, and some mourners use it to explain to others what bereavement and grieving are like for them.

In their turn, those who wish to support and comfort the bereaved tell me that the task-based idea provides them with the understanding that they seek. It enables them to grasp the general shape and contour of the disruption in living that those they care about have experienced and gives them insight into the variety of challenges the bereaved face. Often, it resonates with the caregivers' own prior loss experiences and helps them to see the strong family resemblances among loss experiences in the human condition. They, too, recognize that in coming to terms with life, death, and suffering as they grieve, the bereaved and they alike are engaged not in ordinary problem solving but rather in coming to terms with something they will never fully control, overcome, or solve. In those ways, the ideas help to build empathy and to bridge the distance between caregivers and those they care about.

The Idea Promotes Respect for Individuality

We learn how to live and be ourselves in different places and surrounded by different things and people. No two of us engage in the same pattern of activities, projects, and commitments. No two of our life stories are identical. No two of us remember the same past, live the same present daily life, or share the same expectations, hopes, and dreams for the future. Each of us experiences the world from a distinctive perspective in life circumstances uniquely our own. Because this is so, no two of us experience bereavement in identical ways. Each loss affects us in a particular time and place in our lives, shatters our distinctive daily living patterns, and disrupts our unique life stories. No two of us long for the return of the same person to the same place in a life once shared. In turn, no two of us face the same challenges in moving beyond our grief emotion, putting our lives together, and going on into the next chapters of our life stories. As we grieve, each of us addresses tasks that are uniquely our own. We struggle to find our own ways among the particular things and places that have been left behind. We struggle to find our own places in relation to fellow survivors, the deceased, and, perhaps, God. We struggle with aspects of ourselves and activities, projects, commitments, memories, hopes, and dreams that we have cared about in our own peculiar ways. Because each of us faces unique tasks, no two paths of grieving are identical.

If others are to respect our individuality as we grieve, they must move through the general understanding that the task-based idea of grieving provides to appreciation of such details of our lives. Respect for us as individuals does not come with seeing how we are like everyone else in our grieving. It comes when others see and appreciate how we are coping with specific events and disarray in our distinctive life circumstances, addressing our particular tasks, and walking paths into futures uniquely our own. The task-based idea provides ample clues about the ranges of tasks before us and serves as a basis for dialogue with us. It orients listeners to the all-important details and helps them to hear what so few seem able to hear—the unique stories of bereavement and grieving we each have to tell.

The Idea Addresses the Helplessness of Bereavement

The great strength of the task-based idea of grieving as active coping is that it asserts unequivocally that we are not, or at least need not be, passive and helpless when we are bereaved. True, bereavement is choiceless, and we incline toward helplessness when we feel at the mercy of events that are beyond our control. If we linger in grief emotion or succumb to the attractions of extreme grief, we risk falling into profound helplessness, powerlessness, and even paralysis. But, we can, and must, choose not to linger or succumb. We do not feel helpless when we believe there is room to exercise control in our lives, when there are constructive and meaningful things for us to do and say. We do not feel helpless when we can see a point to leaving passivity behind and actively engaging in life. When we grieve, we can and do control our responses to our losses and give direction to our coping. As we address the tasks of grieving, we have many choices about constructive and meaningful things to do and say. The point of choosing to grieve and addressing the tasks is to put together the pieces of our broken lives and to find ways of living purposefully and meaningfully again. As it stresses that only we can do the work of actively coping, the task-based idea asserts that only we have the power to reshape and redirect our lives. As we do so, we overcome our helplessness.

The Idea Provides Guidance for Caregivers

We are all bereaved at some times in our lives. We then need caregivers who know how to support and comfort us as we grieve. More often, however, we find ourselves in the caregiver role and therefore need some idea about how to support and comfort those we care about as they mourn. I believe that the idea that grieving entails actively addressing tasks suggests much that caregivers can do and say.

As caregivers, we can *help mourners see that grieving is active and that it requires that they meet challenges and address specific tasks.* This in itself can be a revelation. We can help mourners recognize the variety of tasks involved in relearning the world; reassure them that they need not meet all challenges or address all tasks at once; help them focus their attention, pace their coping, and remain in character; and support them as they meet specific challenges, address particular tasks, and try their skills in unique circumstances. As we support mourners, we can listen, suggest, rehearse, motivate and inspire, protect privacy, provide company, debrief, comfort, and console.

We can *support others as they use coping capacities that work well for them.* Respecting their individuality requires that we enable them to remain in character and cope on their own terms and in their own ways, even if their ways differ from ours. Some of us regularly and effectively decide self-reflectively and deliberately; some continue to do so as they grieve. We can help them self-consciously to define alternative grieving paths and sort and evaluate them and support them as they enact their choices. Others among us regularly and effectively give direction to their lives but hardly ever self-reflectively or deliberately. Instead, they straightforwardly, but not self-consciously, act in character from well-established motives, dispositions, intentions, and habits. We can encourage them to trust their own, viable coping patterns, to keep doing what works for them.

We can *support others as they learn how to choose more effectively and find new ways of coping.* Some adults have had little experience in giving direction to their own lives by deciding for themselves. Others merely lack experience in choosing during times of bereavement. We can either encourage them to use the skills they have used effectively in other life settings or support them in learning new coping skills. We can help them all to recognize alternative ways of dealing with things, places, other people, and aspects of themselves. We can encourage those who are ordinarily self-reflective to be so in identifying options as they grieve. We can support them as they sort and evaluate the alternatives. We can encourage and support them as they enact their choices. We can help someone whose coping style is ordinarily not self-reflective by sharing stories of others with similar experiences, histories, and characters who have grieved effectively. Such stories may inspire mourners, show them what others have done and said that might work for them, or evoke new responses from them without requiring that they deliberate self-consciously. We may know such stories from friends, relatives, peers, counselors, literature, or scripture. When such an approach fails, we can encourage those who customarily act without self-reflection or deliberation to try a more self-conscious approach to meeting challenges as they grieve. In effect, we can educate mourners for choice, not by choosing for them but by supporting them as they learn how to choose more effectively for themselves as they grieve.

We can do much to *promote and support development of new coping skills in children*. We can assure children that their needs for food, shelter, and love will be met. We can choose words that they understand as we speak to them and explain in very concrete terms new things that they may see, hear, smell, or touch. We can answer questions honestly and patiently in ways that help orient them to reality and not create or support fantasies, for example about where the dead are or their possible return. After we are sure that they have a solid understanding of the concrete reality of what has happened, we can introduce abstract ideas about a possible afterlife or the like in age-appropriate ways. We can comfort children as they experience feelings for which they lack words and support and encourage nonverbal expression of those feelings, through play, drawing, or crying. We can assure them that their experiences are respected. We can give them choices and help them to find meaningful things to do and say (to address their helplessness). We can communicate trust and build their self-confidence as they choose and give direction to their own lives and grieving. We can assure them that they are not alone but rather grieve as parts of families and communities that embrace them.

As caregivers, *we can support and comfort those with impaired capacities*. We must balance respect for their continuing, albeit diminished, capacities to choose for themselves and their particular limitations. We must recognize that they may feel overwhelmed by their losses. We can help them to see how and where meaningful choice is possible for them. Where it is possible, respect requires that we support it. Where prior to loss of capacity some mourners may have found their own course through bereavement without difficulty, they may now need assistance in seeing alternatives, encouragement to act, and patience and reassurance about self-doubts. As when caring for children, we can assure the impaired that their needs will be met, communicate clearly, explain concretely, answer honestly and counter delusion or fantasy, offer comfort for distressing feelings and support their expression, provide respect, trust them and support their self-confidence, and assure them that they are not alone. When they are not lucid, we can provide such things as physical safety, comfort, consolation, patience, reassurance, and love.

Finally, *we can motivate mourners to resist the attractions of grief and begin to address the tasks of grieving*. Most dying persons I have known express the fervent desire that their survivors not be overcome by their deaths and that they live well in their absence. Typically, they hope not to be forgotten but rather to retain a place in their survivors' lives. Effective grieving makes it possible for mourners to remember without intense pain and anguish and to cherish memories of those they have cared about. Indeed, it is possible for survivors to enjoy a transformed, dynamic, life-affirming, and sustaining relationship with those who die through continued interaction with the story of the life now ended.[20] We can motivate mourners to resist the attractions of grief and instead address the tasks of coping by invoking this powerfully persuasive thought: When we grieve, we must let go of the debilitating desire to have those we have loved restored to life that lies at the heart of the emotion grief. We must cope actively in relearning the world in order to secure for those we have lost a new, vital place in ongoing and meaningful life. As we do so, we fulfill the wishes (most often real and at times imagined) of our loved ones for us and reap the most precious rewards of the labors of our grieving. As C. S. Lewis observed in reflecting on his own grieving;

> And suddenly at the very moment when, so far, I mourned H. least, I remembered her best. . . . It was as if the lifting of the sorrow removed a barrier. . . . Passionate grief does not link us with the dead but cuts us off from them. . . . It is just at those moments when I feel least sorrow. . . that H. rushes on my mind in her full reality, her otherness.

Not, as in my worst moments, all foreshortened and patheticized and solemnized by my miseries, but as she is in her own right.[21]

In choosing to grieve actively, we choose life.

Notes

1. John Bowlby, *Attachment and Loss: Attachment*, vol. 1 (New York: Basic Books, 1969); *Attachment and Loss: Separation: Anxiety and Anger*, vol. 2 (New York: Basic Books, 1973); and *Attachment and Loss: Loss, Sadness and Depression*, vol. 3 (New York: Basic Books, 1980).

2. See Chapter 6 for extensive treatment of this aspect of relearning the world.

3. Erich Lindemann, "Symptomatology and Management of Acute Grief," *American Journal of Psychiatry* 101 (1944): 141–148.

4. John Bowlby, "Processes of Mourning," *International Journal of Psycho-Analysis* 42 (1961): 317–340.

5. George Engel, "Grief and Grieving," *American Journal of Nursing* 64 (1964): 93–98.

6. Colin Murray Parkes, "'Seeking' and 'Finding' a Lost Object: Evidence from Recent Studies of the Reaction to Bereavement," in *Normal and Pathological Responses to Bereavement* (New York: MSS Information Corporation, 1974). First published in *Social Science and Medicine* 4 (1970): 187–201; Bowlby, *Attachment and Loss*, vol. 3.

7. Elisabeth Kubler-Ross, *On Death and Dying* (New York: Macmillan, 1969).

8. Lindemann, "Symptomatology."

9. George Engel, "Is Grief a Disease? A Challenge for Medical Research," *Psychosomatic Medicine* 23 (1964): 18–22.

10. Colin Murray Parkes, *Bereavement: Studies of Grief in Adult Life* (New York: International Universities Press, 1972).

11. Therese Rando, *Treatment of Complicated Mourning* (Champaign, Ill.: Research Press, 1993).

12. Beverly Raphael, *The Anatomy of Bereavement* (New York: Basic Books, 1983).

13. Including Phyllis Silverman and Dennis Klass.

14. True, the ill or injured at times actively contribute to their own recovery. However, the still considerable passivity in healing and recovery from illness and injury do not resemble how we far more actively engage in coming to terms with bereavement.

15. Lindemann, "Symptomatology."

16. Colin Murray Parkes, and Robert Weiss, *Recovery from Bereavement* (New York: Basic Books, 1983).

17. William Worden, *Grief Counseling and Grief Therapy: A Handbook for the Mental Health Practitioner*, 1st ed. (New York: Springer Publishing Company, 1982); 2nd ed. (New York: Springer Publishing Company, 1991). The tasks cited here are from the second edition.

18. The focus falls upon Worden's account for several reasons: It is the most encompassing of the task-based accounts, and it shares the limitations of the other views and, therefore, well represents the type of view in need of refinement. Worden, far more than anyone else known to the author, has built his entire account and program of grief counseling and grief therapy around the view that grieving centrally turns upon addressing such tasks. His view is currently the best known and the most influential among the task-based descriptions, and his views warrant careful scrutiny.

19. Similar correspondences obtain with challenges on Lindemann's and Parkes's lists.

20. See Chapter 6 for elaboration of this idea.

21. C. S. Lewis, *A Grief Observed* (New York: Bantam Books, 1976), pp. 52, 64.

3

Respecting Individuals
When They Grieve

"Vain is the word of a philosopher which does not
heal any suffering of man."

Epicurus

The Story of Bill and Diane

Recall the story of Bill and Diane, whose children, Ann, Mike, and
Jimmy, died in their home along with Diane's sister Mary. Bill and
Diane had taken a second honeymoon weekend vacation and had
left the children with Mary. Diane's mother, Margaret, found the
children and their aunt when they did not respond to her telephone
call and, later, to her knock at the door. Margaret opened a back pa-
tio door, entered the home, and discovered all four dead in upstairs
bedrooms. They had been asphyxiated by gas from an improperly
installed gas fireplace. It appeared to Margaret that Mary had tried to
rouse the children from sleep during the night. She guessed that
Mary had smelled the leak too late to prevent all, including herself,
from succumbing. The scene was tragic and, oddly, both peaceful
and grisly. She never described the scene to either Bill or Diane.

Bill and Diane had built their lives around their family. They
had always wanted many children, having enjoyed childhoods with
several siblings and living still near many members of their extended families. Because Bill and Diane lived so close to Mary, she was
readily available to stay with the children, and it was only natural
that Margaret would check in with them on a quiet morning.

The framework for the thinking in this chapter was first developed in my
"Death, Respect and Vulnerability," in *The Dying Human*, ed. Andre deVries and
Amnon Carmi (Ramat Gan, Israel: Turtledove Press, 1979).

Diane had devoted herself to her children and had chosen to stay home with them while they were young. She anticipated having more children. She delighted in her children's every accomplishment and felt especially creative and fulfilled as she nurtured them and supported their development. She believed that the contributions of devoted parents were underappreciated and considered her work as a mother the world's most important responsibility. She accepted as part of that responsibility the daily chores that others saw as drudgery. She enthusiastically joined the PTA at Ann's school, volunteered her time at Mike's preschool, and sat with children Jimmy's age at Sunday school. She believed that her relationship with Bill came first and was the foundation of a good home for her children. She especially enjoyed the shared responsibility of raising the children and the fulfillment that accompanied the parents' cooperation. She relished her children's laughter and comforted them when they were hurt or ill. Hours flew by each day as she read with and to them, played with them, listened to their stories, and observed the many "firsts" in their lives.

Bill had devoted himself to Diane and the children. He felt well tuned into the rhythms of family life and was eager to find as much time in the evenings and on the weekends as he could to enjoy their company. He, too, played often with the children, read to them, delighted in watching them grow, and especially enjoyed tucking each into bed at night after a bedtime story. As the owner of a successful local business he often was able to come home for lunch with Diane and the children and occasionally took time away from work to attend special events in the children's lives. Although he took pride in his work, he especially valued the fact that it enabled him to provide abundantly for his family. He protected his family, closely supervised construction of the large house they moved into shortly after Ann was born, and took great care to insist that all of the most up-to-date safety measures were built into the house.

Bill and Diane had been recognized as "parents of the year" in their community a year before the accident. Bill seconded the view of many that Diane was a model homemaker and mother, and he was very proud of her. Diane, in her turn, thought Bill an unusually devoted husband and father and welcomed his loving support for her decision to dedicate herself to domestic life. Both appreciated the warm embrace of their extended families and the recognition of their church and the broader community.

The second honeymoon trip was the first time they had left the children for more than a few hours. A friend from the local Rotary

Club had approached Bill early in the week and suggested a retreat to a mountain condominium as fun for them and a fine surprise for their wives. The next day Bill surprised Diane with the tickets. She first hesitated about the children, then arranged for Mary to sit, and finally accepted the romantic gesture. They left at midday on Thursday and enjoyed Friday, spending some time alone and some time with their friends.

Now, late on Saturday morning, Earl, Margaret's husband and Diane's father, calls and surprises them while they are enjoying brunch with their friends. Bill takes the call and is at first pleased, although a bit surprised, to hear Earl's voice. Within moments he hears the most devastating words he has ever heard and simply disintegrates into uncontrollable moaning. He blurts out a barely intelligible version of what he's just heard and hands the phone to Diane. While Diane listens to the same news, Bill pounds his head with his fist and hits his head against the wall. His friends try to no avail to constrain and calm him. Diane, too, is overwhelmed by the terrible news and is quickly reduced to a rush of tears and breathless sobbing. Bill's friend takes the phone and listens to Earl in his own disbelief. As painful as the news is, he retains more of the detail of what happened and later helps Bill and Diane with some of their questions. Fortunately for Bill and Diane, their friends are with them and arrange for them all to return on a flight that afternoon. They pack for them, provide what comfort they can, finally force a tranquilizer on Bill to dampen his fervor for hitting his head, and maintain order in the midst of the chaos that Bill and Diane experience as the complete unraveling of their lives.

Their friends take Bill and Diane to Earl's and Margaret's home. The bodies of their three children and Mary are at the funeral home, and they cannot face, at least now, returning to the scene of the tragedy, their own home, now forever the site of their greatest loss. Only as they enter Diane's parents' home does either Diane or Bill fully realize that Mary, too, has died and that Margaret has witnessed something terrible. Diane weeps anew at the loss of her closest family confidant and one of her best friends, a person she was used to calling on when she needed support. Margaret is sedated and resting fitfully. Neither Bill nor Diane wants to disturb her or to hear what she has to tell.

Their disbelief compels Bill and Diane to demand to be taken to the funeral home to see Ann, Mike, Jimmy, and Mary. The pain of the full confrontation crushes them. Yet both begin to say goodbye to each of the children and to Mary, and their peaceful faces comfort them. The next day they arrange the funeral for their children. The visitation period at the funeral home and the funeral itself attract many people who offer support and condolences. Bill's and Diane's parents and siblings and their extended families mean the most to them, and the sharing of their anguish and the warmth of feeling gratify them.

Still, when they leave the cemetery, Bill and Diane feel devastated and terribly alone. Neither can face returning to their own home, and they gratefully accept the invitation of Diane's brother Jerry to move in with his family for a time. They recognize that they might never wish to, or be able to, return to live in their home. But neither wants to decide immediately. This loss of their home compounds the loss of their children. Within a month they decide not to return to their home because their memories are tainted with the thought of their children's deaths. They decide instead to buy a new home.

They are fortunate to find another place quickly, yet they face the difficult challenge of returning to their first home to sort all that is left there of their own and their children's possessions. Although others offer to go with them, they decline that support and manage to move within three months following the accident. The activity exhausts them but provides odd respite from the otherwise great emptiness of their days. Although he is greatly fatigued and eats only when absolutely necessary, Bill invests great, near-frenetic energy in activity, as he returns to work two weeks after the funeral and loses himself in the details of sorting the contents of their home at night and on the weekends. Diane eats little and becomes quite lethargic, although she manages usually to join Bill on the evenings and weekends at their old home. They make many decisions together about what to discard immediately—what to give to family, friends, or the church; what to hold dear and treasure in their new home; what to set aside to decide about later.

Each seems inconsolable to the other. Diane recognizes the old pattern in Bill as he desperately seeks ways to keep busy and says little about the hurt deep inside. His younger sister, Kim, died when he was sixteen, and Diane senses that he was deeply troubled by that loss and never effectively dealt with his emotions. He has told her that he never cried for Kim, and he seems haunted by feelings of the unfairness of death in youth. Diane is unaware of Bill's frequent visits to the children's graves and the tears he sheds there. Although she says nothing, she fears she might lose him, too. Bill barely tolerates Diane's tears as he tries so hard to keep back his own, and he senses that she is so fragile that she could break at any moment. Her whole life was devoted to the children, and he doesn't know how she will be able to go on without her family. He recognizes in her grief over Mary something of his own pain at losing Kim, but he cannot comfort her. Although he does not say so, he feels he might lose her, too. He so wants to make it all better for both of them and is at a complete loss as to how even to begin. At the very least, each senses that the other can provide little support and hesitates even to ask. Each feels that the other dwells at a painful distance that they may never overcome.

In their anguish, each begins to think of starting a new family, for children seem to be what brought them the greatest happiness. Living without children seems unthinkable, and they renew efforts, begun shortly before the mountain trip, to conceive. Their feelings are profoundly jumbled and ambivalent. The hope is exhilarating; having more children seems a way of escaping the pain. Yet neither is confident he or she can love a new child as much as the three who died. The fear of future loss is palpable. Bill fears that he will again fail to protect his family. Diane knows no other way of parenting yet fears that her nurturing was somehow inadequate or the children would still be alive. The longing to be with their dead children tempts each to think he or she might be better off with them. Still, they want desperately to have more children and to find a way to love them in their own right and not as replacements.

Bill senses that he has become a social misfit. He is uncomfortable with family and friends alike, yet dreads being alone. His own family tends to be silent about the experiences that mean everything to him. Although he would not be comfortable with open discussion, he nevertheless resents what he reads in them as a failure to appreciate how much he hurts. He envies, but is nevertheless uncomfortable with, the more open discussion of the tragedy in Diane's family. Although he appreciates the concern and sympathy of others, his pain does not diminish. Friends from Rotary and other associations, when they do not ignore his grief altogether, offer glib advice that misses the depth of his anguish entirely and borders on insult. He wishes someone could just hold him, rather than shake his hand and utter clichés. He senses that some friends, perhaps reluctantly but nonetheless deeply, blame him for having taken Diane away to play on the weekend of the accident. He no longer feels like himself at work, where people seem to be watching him too closely. He ends his regular church attendance because of both the painful memory of the four caskets on the day of the funeral and a growing disbelief that a good God walks with him. Diane brings him to one meeting of a bereaved parents' support group, but he does not return. There is comfort there, but the exposure is too much for him, at least while his grief seems so fresh and raw. He cannot imagine ever seeking professional help; he thinks he may one day approach his minister, although he hesitates for fear that the minister will not tolerate his questions and intense anger at God.

Diane, too, is ill at ease socially. Sharing grief with her family comforts her somewhat, although she misses acutely Mary's usual support. It hurts her so to see her mother so troubled, and she feels helpless in approaching her. She wants both the comfort her mother is unable to provide and the understanding of her mother's torment that eludes her. The evasive pattern in Bill's family troubles her. Several friends listen well in private conversation, but she misses the good times they formerly enjoyed as couples. She misses the interaction with others at schools and at church. She finds the bereaved parents' support group very helpful, determines to continue attending by herself, and hopes eventually to persuade Bill to return with her. She suspects she may need professional help, and she is not reluctant to entertain that thought seriously.

Bill is not comfortable with introspection, and the pain of realizing how much he had taken for granted in life with the children nearly overwhelms him when he dwells in it. It is not that he ignores the feelings; rather, he deals with them most effectively by engaging in activity that constructively reorients him in the world changed radically by the deaths. Diane is far more comfortable probing her feelings. Though her growing awareness of how much she, like Bill, had taken for granted in life is painful for her, the pain does not paralyze her. Instead, she uses her growing self-awareness to discern what she needs to do self-consciously to forge ahead in life without those who have died.

Margaret feels isolated in her grief. She has lost both a daughter and three precious grandchildren. Her daughter Diane and her son-in-law Bill seem hurt beyond words, and she wonders if they will enjoy life ever again. She appreciates their desire for a child, worries that they are not ready, and bites her tongue. She knows she will never tell them of the sight of their children or of her daughter who died with them. She tries to tell Earl, but he insists that it is best not to speak of such things and to go on as if they had never happened. The scene replays in her mind endlessly. She tries to hide her agitation from Earl for fear of upsetting his heart, weakened by a heart attack three years before the accident. However, she cannot clear her mind of the scene while lying next to him at night. When he drifts into sleep, she walks the floor alone. She ordinarily works her way through difficulty in her life in a very businesslike, no-nonsense manner, but this pattern fails her in her current distress. She senses that she needs help and thinks she will approach her minister soon.

Respecting Individual Ways of Flourishing

Life was wonderful for Bill, Diane, and Margaret. Then, when they expected it least, it became awful. If we are to respect them as the unique individuals they are, we must appreciate how they lived and flourished before the loss of so much of what they had taken for granted. Only then can we appreciate what and how they have lost. We need to understand the shape of each of their life patterns and the places that caring about and for Ann, Mike, Jimmy, and Mary held in each of their lives. What was it like for them to share daily life with those who died? What had each come to expect as their daily routines revolved around or included them? What did they do and experience with them that brought satisfaction, fulfillment, reward, a sense of purpose or meaning? How were the stories of their lives entangled with the stories of the lives now ended? How had they changed each in his or her own way for knowing and living with them? What were their hopes and dreams for the futures they expected to share with them?

If we are to respect the individuality of those who are grieving, we must understand and appreciate the details of their lives before bereavement. How did they flourish while those now dead were with them? What did they do with and for those who died? How did sharing life with them color and shape their experiences? How did they interweave their lives with those now ended in ways they found meaningful?

We Find Meaning in Activity

Before he married, Bill took great pride in his work, first as a craftsman and then as owner of his own contracting business. He never lost his love for working with his hands and for making things that last. He worked long hours, saved his money, and struck out on his own. His management skills matched his skills with his hands, and his firm prospered. Still, independent life was not enough. He joined the Rotary Club and found satisfaction in community service. But nothing matched the joy that he found in his marriage and in supporting

Diane and their young children. It seemed then that his work took on new meaning. He watched over his family, provided abundantly for them, and devoted much of his leisure time to special projects at home. He was especially careful to make sure that when their house was built, the finest materials were used and every safety measure was taken.

Diane never found much satisfaction in the jobs she took after high school. She worked to live, not the other way around. Her mother, Margaret, appeared to have had a wonderful life; like her, Diane always wanted marriage and a large family. She was determined to marry only when she found a man whom she loved and respected and who returned those feelings and one she believed would be a loving father. In Bill she found all she had ever hoped for. She delighted in making a home and in day-to-day domestic life with him. She found her greatest fulfillment in giving birth to Ann, Mike, and Jimmy and nurturing them with Bill at her side. She could imagine no more important creative activity, and she resented those who suggested that she had somehow settled for second best in not pursuing a career outside the home. That was all right for some, but it wasn't for her. She believed that she was meant to be a wife and a mother. Her volunteer service at the church and her children's schools seemed a natural extension of that calling.

Margaret, too, experienced great satisfaction as she raised her large family and cared for her husband, Earl. Although she did not enjoy the full cooperation and participation at home that Diane enjoyed with Bill, she nevertheless thrived in her thoroughly domestic roles. She took pride in her children's accomplishments and was especially gratified when they, too, wanted large families. When she was presented with grandchildren, she accepted as many invitations from Diane to help as time permitted.

In order to respect Bill, Diane, Margaret, or any one who is grieving, we must learn how their activities have given meaning to their lives. We flourish as persons as we realize what Victor Frankl has called achievement values;[1] that is, we find meaning in *doing* things as we pursue purposes we deem worthy; make contributions to our families, friends, or broader communities; make or create things; use our talents; accomplish and achieve; and make a difference while we are here. We define our individuality, in part, as we adopt unique patterns of daily activity and take on projects that become major themes in our life stories.

The range of ways in which we experience ourselves as achieving, contributing, and making important differences through what we do is almost as broad and as richly varied as human activity itself. Respecting any of us requires that others learn how we find meaning in activities. Some of us derive satisfaction and fulfillment from work outside the home as we put in a good day's work at the office or factory, perform assigned tasks reliably and faithfully, make a product to specifications, finish an assignment on time, refine a process or technique, learn and use skills, invent new products and processes, make a suggestion for change and have it accepted, establish a business, offer professional services, teach, counsel, manage, lead, foster cooperative effort and team spirit, or provide for a family. Some of us find satisfaction and fulfillment in domestic life as we put in a good day's work at home, nurture a child's development, make a child, spouse, or companion happy, mediate disputes, maintain a household, cook, protect loved ones, support others in times of crisis, or care for the sick and the elderly. Some of us find purpose and meaning in building relationships in the broader community as we give through friendship, bring a smile or comfort to those who are less well off, share talents through volunteer or community service, support charities, join worthy causes, or pursue political objectives. Many of us derive satisfaction and fulfillment from creative or leisure activity as we make things with our hands, create artistically, sing, dance, play a musical instrument, exercise and care for our bodies, or participate in sports. And many of us find mental and spiritual satisfaction and fulfillment as we think creatively, seek solutions to problems, contemplate, meditate, pray, and pursue personal and spiritual growth. No two of us fill our days with the same activities or find the identical satisfaction, fulfillment, purpose or meaning in them.

We Find Meaning in Experiences

Bill treasured innumerable experiences with his wife and children. He knew a vibrant and joyful closeness with Diane. Knowing and being known by her gladdened his heart, and he knew a rare peace and comfort. Through Diane's influence, he grew personally as he gave voice to tenderness and nurturing that he never expressed before. He often expressed his appreciation to her for all she had given him. He attended the birth of each child. Hours of play with Ann, Mike, and Jimmy together and with each separately brought much delight and pleasure into his life. Reading to the children and hearing their stories filled his heart.

Diane, too, experienced her marital and family life as rich

and rewarding. Bill's affection, imaginative flair, and devotion often touched and delighted her. Through Bill's influence and as others recognized her for her hours of volunteer service, she grew in self-reliance and self-esteem. The births of Ann, Mike, and Jimmy high-lighted her life. Nursing each child brought closeness and treasured memories. She cherished their smiles, hugs, laughter, drawings, and school projects. She was grateful simply to have been alive to see and share so many "firsts" in each of their lives. She knew as well the confidences, love, and affection of her dear sister Mary.

Margaret, through the years, knew loving and being loved by Earl, their children, and their children's children. Although life was not always hearts and roses, her joys and delights were abundant. Like her daughter Diane and her son-in-law Bill, she believed in God and at times experienced herself as meaningfully touched by his grace.

In order to respect Bill, Diane, Margaret, or any one who is griev-ing, we must learn how their experiences have helped them to be-lieve that their lives are worthwhile. We flourish as we realize what Frankl has called experiential values,[2] finding meaning in *experienc-ing* things we value either as we look within ourselves, interact with others (especially in love relationships), enjoy the fruits of culture, dwell in our natural surroundings, or commune with the divine. Either at the time of the experiences or on later reflection we per-ceive that the experiences have contributed to the worth and mean-ing of our lives. We are grateful that we have lived to know the experience, to be fulfilled in or satisfied by it. We find our individual-ity, in part, as we live distinctive life histories and flourish in, and accumulate memories of, unique combinations of such experiences.

The range of ways in which we perceive ourselves as fulfilled, satisfied, or living meaningfully through what we experience is al-most as broad and richly varied as human experience itself. Some of us derive satisfaction and fulfillment from such things as the plea-sures, satisfactions, and fulfillment of physical exertion or perfor-mance, laughter, the senses, physical and emotional intimacy, insight and wisdom, flights and expressions of imagination, person-al growth and development, and personal autonomy. Some of us find meaning in interaction with others as we experience such things as recognition and reward, acceptance and forgiveness, affection, close-ness and companionship, good conversation, shared moments of excitement and joy, celebrations, or others' thoughtfulness or gener-osity. Some of us derive satisfaction or fulfillment in our cultural surroundings as we experience such things as community or historic events, a good story, music, painting or sculpture, dramatic performance, or sports thrills. Some of us find meaning in our natural surroundings as we experience such things as the delights of camping beneath the stars or fishing in a quiet lake, the grandeur of a mountain or a forest, the order in a coastal wetland, the roar of a storm at sea, the beauty of a sunset, the intricacy of a spider's web, the majesty of a soaring eagle, or the awesome power of a polar bear. Some of us find spiritual meaning as we experience such things as reverence before God and creation, the embrace of divine grace, perseverance through trial, or divine forgiveness and acceptance. No two of us fill our days with the same experiences or find the identical satisfaction, fulfillment, purpose, or meaning in them.

We Find Meaning Through Connection

Bill could not believe how good it felt to be a husband and father. Even those things that he had found rewarding when he was single seemed at least doubled in their significance. He wasn't just working for his own satisfaction or comfort; his work enabled him to provide support, comfort, and security for Diane and the children. He loved deeply and was loved in return. Diane was his best friend and his life's companion as well as his wife. She drew from him a tender strength he never knew he had. He enjoyed nothing more than building memories with her, sharing daily life, and hoping and dreaming about the future. His days were filled with surprises and unforgettable moments of shared experience. Each child held a special place in his heart. Ann's loving eyes melted his heart. Mike's irrepressible giggle nearly always signaled that he was hiding some recent mischief. Jimmy's arms would not loose their grip when Bill brought him to bed. Quiet times as he read each a story before sleep were the best moments, each in its own way. As he helped Diane at home, he looked toward a future where Ann, Mike, and Jimmy would be adults with children of their own. As he began to show Ann and Mike how to play baseball, fish, and enjoy the outdoors (and anticipated doing the same with Jimmy), he felt the way he thought his own father must have felt before him. He sensed that he would walk with his children even after he died.

Diane found what she had always wanted when she married Bill and started her family. Single life had seemed somehow selfish to her. In marriage she gave so much and, she believed, received so much in return. Sharing domestic labors with Bill added to their meaning. She told him often how grateful she was for the comfort, security, and love that he provided for her and the children. She felt close to her mother as she sought her advice and sensed that she was following the same path through life that her mother had chosen. Nurturing her children seemed to her the most important calling possible. Indeed, she believed it to be God's work. But it wasn't just labor. As with Bill, each child held a special place in her heart. When Ann began imitating her every move, Diane looked toward the day when Ann in her turn would raise children. When Mike, having hurt himself, would come to her for care and comfort, she repaired the damage, held him close, then held her breath as he sallied forth again. Jimmy stayed closer to her, and she relished every smile as he shared all of his discoveries. She felt that her love for children was unbounded and eagerly anticipated bringing still more children into the world with Bill at her side. In the meantime, she reached other children through her volunteer work at Ann's school and at the church. She maintained a closeness to Mary that only sisters know, calling her often and watching their children together.

Margaret found her greatest fulfillment as wife to Earl, mother to Diane, Mary, and her other children, and grandmother to so many, including Ann, Mike, and Jimmy. Each loved one held a special place in her heart and was part of the amazing living quilt she thought her family to be. Nothing mattered as much to her as her family's health and well-being. Mary had been a frail child, and Margaret had spent long, anxious nights bringing her through lingering fevers. It was thus especially gratifying to see Mary thriving as an adult with a young family of her own. Margaret admired Diane for standing by Mary as a child and was pleased to see how close they remained as adults. Margaret delighted in planning for holidays, birthdays, anniversaries, and countless special occasions. She gave generously, with no expectation of return. She felt profoundly grateful to God for giving her the opportunity to start something so grand, to witness its unfolding, and to sense that her family would continue to flourish long after she and Earl had gone. She felt as she believed so many other mothers must have felt before her—at home in a mysterious but doubtless grand scheme of things.

In order to respect Bill, Diane, Margaret, or anyone who is grieving, we must learn how connections with others or something greater than themselves has given meaning to their lives. Through such *connections* we sense that we live in the service of a higher purpose, have a reason to live, leave the world a better place for having been here, and find a place in a larger history or scheme of things. Within complex, often rich, and inevitably unique and idiosyncratic life patterns, we share life with others. Each individual life pattern is like a tapestry of interwoven threads of experience, achievement, caring, and connection. Our life tapestries take on unique shapes, textures, and colors, in part as a function of the variety of connections we make and experience, and this interweaving of threads of connection importantly defines who we are.[3]

We find some activities and experiences especially meaningful as they enable us to feel connected to something transcendent, something greater than ourselves. While we experience some *achievements* as significant only for ourselves, for example, reaching a new plateau in physical fitness or gaining hard-won insight into our own limitations, we experience other achievements as having significance beyond ourselves or as contributing something of lasting value, for example, guiding our children, creating a work of art, serving others well on the job, or volunteering for community service. Similarly, we perceive some *experiences* as significant only for ourselves—enjoying a hearty laugh or delighting in a flight of fancy. Yet we value other experiences as in them we realize connectedness to such things as our friends, family, the community, a heritage or tradition, a cause, nature, God, the future after we have gone, or an afterlife. We may sense this connectedness when we enjoy a reunion with friends, listen to the sorrows of a family member, serve on a school board, feel continuities with our parents, join in ritual celebrations, devote energies to cleaning the environment for those to come after, feel the closeness of God in church or in the mountains, provide for our children and grandchildren, or anticipate seeing those who have died before us. No two of us weave identical patterns of connection in the world or find the same satisfaction, fulfillment, purpose, or meaning in them.

Respecting Individual Vulnerabilities

As we come to understand and appreciate how Bill, Diane, and Margaret shaped their lives to include caring about and for Ann, Mike, Jimmy, and Mary, we learn how each was vulnerable to hurting in his or her own unique ways when they died. If we are to respect them, or any among us, as the individuals they are in their times of loss, we must appreciate their distinctive vulnerabilities. Each of us suffers uniquely because each of us is vulnerable to the shattering of a particular life pattern and the disruption of a particular life story. When we are bereaved, we experience the pain of loss as the taken-for-granted pattern of caring for and about, and flourishing with, those who have died is halted abruptly. The time and effort we spend in grieving disrupts and distorts other taken-for-granted patterns of caring and flourishing in the broader context of our lives. Each of us faces a unique combination of challenges and must address tasks uniquely our own in grieving. Our flourishing as the individuals we are is in crisis, and how we grieve decisively influences our future flourishing and who we become. As we grieve, we learn to flourish again in the absence of those who have died.

Our vulnerability in bereavement does not stop with the shattering of our life patterns and disruption of our life stories. We are also vulnerable to factors that may interfere with, hinder, compromise, undermine, inhibit, or even stifle our coping effectively. Such factors frustrate our attempts to establish a transformed pattern of caring and flourishing and again live meaningfully and purposefully.

We Are Vulnerable in Our Connections with Those Who Die

The loss of a single child requires survivors to meet challenges presented by nearly the full range of objects, things, places, events, and relationships in the worlds of their experience, since few of these remain untouched by the relationship with the child. Bill's and Diane's multiple losses tragically compound these challenges. The home they once shared with Ann, Mike, and Jimmy is so filled with painful reminders that they choose not to return to it. In doing so they incur the secondary loss of that home and all it means to them. They sort the contents of the home in often painful encounters. They set aside some favorite toys and clothing for later disposition. For now it is too painful either to part with them or to face them. The town where they live, too, is filled with difficult places. Once-happy holidays, birthdays, and anniversaries are now dreadful. The losses affect virtually every relationship in their families, with friends, and in the broader community, especially those with each other, Margaret, Mary's husband, Chris (tinged with guilt because they had asked Mary to stay with their children), and Chris's three children (who remind them of their own losses).

The variety of items that carry memories of her grandchildren is not as extensive for Margaret as it is for Bill and Diane, since her grandchildren did not share her home. Still, special objects and places in her home and elsewhere present difficulties. She loves the photos and gifts they gave and made for her, but she can barely stand to look at them. Moreover, she grieves as a mother. Her home, which had sheltered Mary before her marriage to Chris ten years earlier, is tinged with memories, especially a guest room (still decorated much as Mary had left it) and, again, the photos. The glorious and frequent extended family gatherings, especially at the holidays, will never be the same. Her relationships with Earl (given his intolerance for her grieving), Bill and Diane (given what she has witnessed but chooses not to tell them), her son-in-law Chris, and Mary's children present the greatest challenges. Her faith is shaken but not broken.

As it is for Bill, Diane, and Margaret, the more connection to the deceased is interwoven in the tapestry of our lives, the greater our vulnerability to having to reweave the fabric. We are burdened differently by the tasks of grieving depending on how our relationships with the deceased gave meaning to our lives. Until we reweave new life patterns and redefine our hopes and aspirations for the future, our flourishing remains diminished. Respecting any of us when we grieve requires understanding the peculiarities and detailed contours of the reweaving required, the specifics of the tasks before us.[4]

We Are Vulnerable to Loss of Wholeness

Both Bill and Diane suffer intensely from a loss of wholeness; very little remains viable of the daily routines that were intricately interwoven with the lives of their children. Their life patterns have been shattered. Diane spent most hours of each day nurturing one or all of them. Bill spent most hours working primarily to provide for them and found evenings, weekends, and occasional escapes from work with them the richest part of his weekly routine. Virtually all of the taken-for-granted perceptions, feelings, desires, motivations, dispositions, and habits that were viable when the children lived are still present but without their usual objects.

Internally, Bill and Diane are in chaos. Incoherence and ambivalence abound. Each partner wants to share his or her grief with the other, yet hesitates to compound the other's burdens. They cherish the memories of life in their home, yet recoil at images of what must have happened there. Bill busies himself at work but finds he is not himself there. He is uncomfortable with others, yet dreads being alone. He understands the pain of losing a sister, yet cannot comfort his wife about losing Mary. He finds comfort in the support group, yet feels the exposure is too much to bear. Diane appreciates the romantic gesture of the second honeymoon but feels guilty about accepting Bill's invitation. She wants her mother's comfort, yet does not seek it. She senses her mother's anguish, yet does not approach to comfort her. The realization that she always confided in Mary tempers her gratitude for her surviving brothers' and sisters' support.

Having so strongly identified themselves as mother and home-maker and as protector and provider for the family, respectively, Diane and Bill feel profoundly incomplete and wonder how the narratives of their lives can possibly end meaningfully. They desire a new family, and yet with the exhilarating hope comes palpable fear of losing again. They long to love new children in their own right but wonder whether they might treat them as replacements. They find it difficult to be hopeful that the future offers any realistic prospect of happiness, and the point of going on is obscure.

Bill entertains thoughts of joining his children in death rather than enduring the separation, finds his work diverting but no longer purposeful, perceives the world as no longer a safe and trustworthy home, and senses that he has been abandoned by God. Diane aches because of the separation from the children and her sister, senses the strain in her relations with her mother and with her brother-in-law's family, cannot imagine returning to volunteer service at the school or Sunday school, distrusts the world as unsafe and threatening, and wonders how God could allow such a thing to happen to one so devoted to her family.

Margaret, too, suffers loss of wholeness. Her regular daily routine was not as intimately interwoven with the lives of Ann, Mike, and Jimmy or with that of Mary as it had once been, yet interaction with her children and grandchildren held a prominent place. Her agitation and restlessness profoundly disrupt and distract her from her daily functioning. Missing those who have died preoccupies her. She is not as wholly invested in her surviving children and grand-children as she was formerly. Life with Earl has changed considerably, given his refusal to hear what she has to tell. She is ambivalent about Earl, both not wanting to upset him and resenting his advice to swallow her grief. She wants to warn Bill and Diane about having other children too soon but holds her tongue, in part because she knows how much children mean to them. She does not feel as profoundly the incompleteness or loss of meaning and purpose in her life. Taken as a whole, her life still seems to her to have been full and rich. Yet, she is so troubled by the haunting vision of the death scene that she fears she may never know peace until she dies. This loss of hope represents a terrible rewriting of the ending of her autobiography, and she wishes at times she had never lived to see it turn out so. She feels disconnected in her now-strained relationships with Earl, Bill, and Diane. She refuses to believe that God intends such things to happen, and she finds what comfort she does in an abiding faith.

Like Bill, Diane, and Margaret, when bereaved we are vulnerable to experiencing our selves as no longer whole as we were when the deceased lived. Respect for any of us when we grieve requires that others appreciate our struggle to be whole again without the deceased. *Loss sunders the coherence of our present living patterns.* We suffer more or less profound disorientation as daily routines once interwoven with those of the deceased lose viability. Internally, our perceptions, feelings, desires, motivations, dispositions, and habits are in disarray. Chaos and disharmony, dissonance, ambivalence, tension, and incoherence abound. *We experience our lives as incomplete* as the death interrupts the unfolding narrative of our life stories. It breaks the expected continuity of past, present, and future. As it affects more or less profoundly the purposes that formerly defined our hopes for the future, it leaves us more or less at a loss as to how meaningfully to continue our autobiographies. *We experience ourselves as disconnected, as parts apart from the wholes within which we find life meaningful.* Most centrally, death separates us from the deceased. Tensions and strains in other relationships heighten our sense of disconnection, of isolation and alienation from community. Some of us experience ourselves as no longer at home in the world and the world itself as unsafe, untrustworthy, and even threatening or frightening. Some of us feel betrayed by the powers or forces of the universe, abandoned by God.

We Are Vulnerable to Anguish over Unfinished Business

The children's deaths nearly overwhelm Bill and Diane in part because of the extent of the unfinished business with them. Raising and experiencing the world with Ann, Mike, and Jimmy was the central business of their lives. Ann lived long enough to speak of what she wanted to do and be "when I grow up." Diane looked forward to leading her through childhood and adolescence toward realizing those barely formulated aspirations and flourishing as a hopeful young woman. She tasted the closeness that only a mother and a daughter can know. Mike's look to the future seemed only fantasy. Yet Bill and Diane saw in him so much potential, and his gentle, caring disposition led each to believe he would become a remarkable young man. Bill introduced both Ann and Mike to activities he anticipated enjoying with them for years to come, and his pride in his children's very early accomplishments burst within him, nightly conversation at bedtime built special father-and-son and father-and-daughter bonds. Diane tasted the closeness that only a mother and a son can know as she tempered Mike's energy with gentleness. Jimmy, barely two, spoke but a few words, and Bill and Diane hadn't a clue as to whom he might become or aspire to be. His personality was emerging already, and he was a delightful child to be with, but both parents feel deprived of the chance really to know him. Bill and Diane are confident that their children knew that their parents loved them, and they have no regrets about words of love and other gestures left unspoken or undone. Still, both are miserable as they realize the difference between the good-byes they said as they left for their trip and those they wish they could now say.

Margaret looked forward to knowing her grandchildren better, sharing their delight in accomplishment, experiencing the world with them as grandmothers do, and lavishing affection on them. She knew and admired Mary as a fine young woman and treasured the mature friendship they had found in recent years. Still, Mary's life seems to have been cut short before she could become all she could be. Margaret laments not seeing Mary's full blossoming, sharing in raising her children, and walking the world with her in her adult years. She, too, is confident that her grandchildren and daughter knew well that she loved them dearly, and she has no regrets over words of love and other gestures left unspoken or undone. Still, she wishes she could hold Mary and her grandchildren one more time.

Like Bill, Diane, and Margaret, we are vulnerable to anguish over lost opportunities to complete unfinished business with the deceased. Most commonly, we long to share anticipated experiences, realize hopes and aspirations for accomplishing something together, utter unspoken words of love and affection, and say good-byes. When adults die, the intensity of our anguish depends on our closeness to, and the extent of our interaction with, the deceased. When children die (no matter their ages), parents realize they can no longer watch and nurture their development. Their very lives seem unfinished when they die prematurely.

We Are Vulnerable to the Lingering Effects of Hurtful Relationships with Those Who Die

Unfortunately, not all of our relationships with those who die are as uncomplicatedly loving as those in our story. When we are bereaved, we are vulnerable to complications in grieving that derive from hurtful or dysfunctional aspects of relationships with the deceased, such as unresolved anger, ambivalence, guilt, or dependence.[5] Some people expect that the loss of relationships that were less than fully loving is less difficult to come to terms with. However, coping with loss where strong negative feelings linger often challenges us unexpectedly. Negative ties are ties as much as are positive ones. Often they bind us more tightly. Our negative feelings persist as we grieve, and our inability to express or resolve them in interaction with the deceased frustrates us. Some of us feel guilty as we harbor these negative feelings and leave them unresolved. Negative treatment and, possibly, abuse at the hands of the deceased continue to undermine our self-esteem, self-confidence, and functioning in relationships with others. Some of us resent the persistent destructive consequences of the relationship on our current life patterns and are so bound by our inability to forgive that we are unable to return to meaningful living as survivors. Loosening such bonds is often profoundly complicated, and we may need the intervention of a trained professional when we cannot free ourselves.[6] Fortunately, Bill, Diane, and Margaret know none of this torment in their bereavement, although it is possible that Margaret would if Earl were to die.

Sometimes we feel guilty toward the deceased for having mistreated or in some way failed them. Imagine, for instance, a father who keeps a gun at home, only to have his child kill himself accidentally with the weapon.[7] Death closes his usual avenues toward reconciliation or forgiveness. When any of us perceives ourself as in any way responsible for the death, the guilt can be excruciating. Tragically, we often are responsible, although rarely entirely so. Bill feels that he failed adequately to protect his family as he supervised the installation of the fireplace insert, but recognition that others did the actual work and did so improperly and that he had done so much for so many years to protect his family mitigates his guilt. Diane wonders what might have happened had she not consented to leave with Bill for the weekend. Confidence that, as she raised her children, she had done her best to provide for and love them mitigates her guilt.

Dysfunctional dependence on the deceased and incomplete or arrested development of the capacity to function autonomously can compromise effective coping. By extension, it can be devastating to lose the sense of purpose in life that derives from meeting the needs of those who depend on us. Parents like Bill and Diane are vulnerable to such loss when their children die. When we have insisted on inappropriate dependence in the deceased, we may feel guilt for having done so.

Negative bonding with the deceased complicates our coming to terms with the emotion grief, especially in its extreme form.[8] We then long for the deceased differently. Our desire is not exclusively loving and affectionate; resentment, frustration, and bitterness are likely to prevail and can bind us strongly. This kind of unfinished business challenges us profoundly. We struggle even to recognize or acknowledge these negative elements in our relationships with the deceased. Even when we do acknowledge them, we often cannot effectively express or come to terms with them. Moreover, strong family and social pressures often reinforce our reluctance to acknowledge, express, and come to terms with negative bonding. Yet unless we do so, the hopeless longing for the deceased will persist.

We Are Vulnerable to "Disenfranchised" Grieving

Margaret tastes an unfortunately too common dismissal of the significance of her grieving. In part, the horror of the triple death of her grandchildren distracts attention from and marginalizes her loss of Mary. No one recognizes that, as Margaret experiences it, Mary's death, even as an adult, still represents the death of the little girl Margaret once nursed at her breast and protected fiercely. It is as if the others think that, because age brings more extensive experience with death and loss, Margaret has a kind of immunity to intense grieving over the loss of her child.

Like Margaret, when we are bereaved, we may experience ourselves as "disenfranchised" in our grieving because something about our relationship with the deceased leads others to fail to recognize our grieving or to stigmatize or dismiss it as illegitimate.[9] Few if any recognize the grieving itself of the parents of adult children, very elderly persons, young children, or retarded, demented, or otherwise mentally compromised individuals. In some instances people dismiss the significance of our relationships with the deceased or discount the value of what is lost, as we lose homosexual partners, extramarital heterosexual partners, stillborns,[10] miscarried or aborted fetuses, loved ones who are severely afflicted or handicapped, pets, prisoners (who are one and all our children, siblings, parents, or spouses), coworkers, public figures, or people from our past, including former spouses, companions, and friends. Sometimes, there is something repugnant about the death, as when those we care about commit suicide,[11] are murdered, or suffer violent or mutilating deaths. Unwillingness to acknowledge our hurt, lack of social support, or even sanction compound the challenges we face in grieving as they add secondary losses; intensify our feelings of abandonment, alienation, guilt and shame, anger, depression, and meaninglessness; and exclude us from social responses to death such as funerals.

We Are Vulnerable Because of the Circumstances of Some Deaths

Bill and Diane lose not one but three children, their entire family. The enormity of the loss stretches the limits of their comprehension. All of the deaths are sudden, unexpected, and traumatic. Although they see the reality of the consequences of the accident when they go to the funeral home, it seems not real that they had just two days before seen their family members with smiling faces and had hugged and kissed them good-bye. Bill and Diane can only imagine the horror of the death scene that Margaret discovered. They choose to live with what they imagine vividly rather than with what she could tell them. Diane often ruminates about whether and how much her children and her sister suffered. The feeling that in some way the deaths were all preventable plagues them as each feels to some extent responsible, yet recognizes that the primary responsibility rests elsewhere. Taking legal action against the fireplace insert installer and possibly against the manufacturer, regardless of whether such action is justified, may distract them from addressing the tasks of grieving. The publicity attendant to the losses complicates their daily living, invades their privacy, and distracts them from coping. A suit and a trial could do more of the same.

Margaret loses not only her daughter Mary but three grandchildren. She struggles with the trauma of coming onto the death scene with no expectation of what she would find. The vision of what she saw haunts her. She fears not being able to escape a comparable accident. The vision and the fear together rob her of her sleep as she walks the floor alone after Earl has fallen asleep. She is especially troubled by her inability to clear her mind of that scene in order to recall how those she loved looked when they were alive. She feels robbed of so many precious memories by this intrusive horror.

Like Bill, Diane, and Margaret, we may find our grieving complicated by the distinctive character of some deaths.[12] Sudden and unexpected deaths heighten surprise, intensify shock and numbness, startle us into realizing how we took the relationship with the deceased for granted, and leave us with more business unfinished. Some of us find if difficult to take in the reality of such losses. Violent, mutilating, or random deaths shock, horrify, and traumatize us in ways that interfere with the usual grieving processes. When we witness such deaths, this interference is exacerbated, and we face the added challenges of posttraumatic stress syndrome (for example, hypervigilance, hypersensitivity to stimuli, nightmares, and fixating visions). When we perceive deaths as preventable or caused by human action or neglect, we frequently are distracted from normal grieving as we preoccupy ourselves with those responsible and adjust to a world we now perceive as threatening, menacing, and untrustworthy. Deaths that follow lengthy illness can exhaust or numb us and leave us with little energy for grieving. We may even expect that our grieving is done when it is only beginning. Deaths of children make us doubt our identities as parents, intensify our feelings of purposelessness and guilt, and often lead us to a belief that there is no fairness in the order of things.

We Are Vulnerable to Limits in Our Coping Capacities

Bill, Diane, and Margaret all face emotional and psychological challenges that test the limits of their coping capacities. Bill does not sort and recognize his emotions well. They frighten him. He retreats from and avoids dealing with them, losing himself instead in activity. He cries freely in private, but his repertoire for expressing his emotions is limited. His ability to carry on day to day and to sort the contents of his home may or may not indicate that he has a high tolerance for carrying his emotions. Carry them he must until he finds effective means to acknowledge, identify, express, and come to terms with them. More than likely, he is avoiding the emotional challenges as he did years earlier when his sister Kim died. He has known success outside the home, yet much of his self-confidence and self-esteem are derived from his success as a parent, and he wonders who he is if not father and protector of his family.

Diane far more ably sorts and recognizes her emotions. They frighten her, too, but she does not retreat. She expresses them fully and freely to whomever will listen. She is, however, more emotionally fragile than Bill, and her lethargy and her inability to sustain the sorting activity with Bill's persistence likely reflect this. Her self-confidence and her sense of worth have derived even more exclusively than his from her success as a parent, and any sense of identity beyond the role of mother eludes her.

Margaret recognizes her emotions only too well. She does not lack motivation or ability to express them effectively. The trauma of what she has seen heightens her sensitivity to emotion, and she nearly bursts with emotional overload. However, because she is reluctant to hurt others or to seek help outside the family, she stifles her own emotional expression. She knows no private or nonverbal modes of expression. Her condition is very much like that of one who suffers from posttraumatic shock disorder, and the tension in her builds toward crisis. Her self-esteem and her sense of identity are strong and intact, but the emotional pressure withers her self-confidence.

Bill and Diane are vulnerable to intensified separation anxiety. Young children who lose a parent when they are testing the safety of independent forays into the world and the reliability of bonds with their parents predictably struggle with separation anxiety following the loss. Parents experience similar separation anxiety when young children die. Having ventured away from their children for the first time that weekend in the mountains, they may experience heightened anxiety in the aftermath of the tragedy.

Like Bill, Diane, and Margaret, we are vulnerable in the limitations of our abilities to cope *emotionally*. Some of us simply are better prepared than others for the psychological and emotional challenges of dealing with loss. Some of us better identify our own emotional responses to loss. Some are more highly motivated to face and address the emotional challenges. Some more effectively meet the challenges and constructively express their emotions (verbally or nonverbally); some come to bereavement with greater self-confidence, higher self-esteem, and more stable identities. As we reach or exceed our emotional limits, however, the onslaught may overwhelm us, induce psychological numbness, or drive us to use psychological defense mechanisms to protect ourselves. Some of us may simply cease altogether coping emotionally or psychologically. This shutdown, in turn, may undermine our effectiveness in other facets of our coping. Emotional fragility, unusual sensitivity, weak self-confidence, low self-esteem, unstable identity, or preexisting psychological or emotional conditions such as separation anxiety, depression or mental illness complicate our grieving. Finally, some of us are more capable than others of overcoming the potentially debilitating extreme grief emotion.[13]

Instinctively, Bill sorts the contents of his house, senses that it is important, but does not grasp self-consciously how it speaks directly to his helplessness in a world out of control. Diane goes along to be with him as long as she can, likewise unaware of the significance of the activity and by disposition more passive. Extreme grief attracts both, and they fantasize regularly about reuniting soon with their children. Only their strong belief that suicide is a sin keeps them from bringing about their own deaths and helps them resist the potentially paralyzing longing for the children's return. As they effectively sort the contents of their home and decide to build a new one, they show that they can conceive of alternatives in dealing with some elements in their lives, evaluate them, and act constructively. However, neither Bill nor Diane imagines a viable, happy daily life without children. This limited adaptability strongly inclines them to conceive again and to risk the possible complications of treating new children as replacements. Bill inclines toward evasion of some of the tasks before him, for example, as he loses himself in his work, keeps busy to the point of near exhaustion, and stifles his expression of emotion and spiritual despair. Diane uses fewer coping strategies that tend to fail, but she is not as accustomed to autonomy as Bill is.

Margaret ordinarily "gets right in there, picks up the pieces, and moves on." However, fixation on the death scene short-circuits her usually active coping pattern. Ordinarily very self-confident, she is surprised at the intensity of the fear and anxiety aroused by the vision of the death scene. She fears that she will never enjoy daily activities again, including visiting with the surviving family members.

Like Bill, Diane, and Margaret, we are vulnerable in the limitations of our abilities to cope *behaviorally*. Grieving requires effort, as well as time. Some of us are more passive than active by disposition. Most of us, as we suffer, remain passive and tied to a known path (even if it is no longer viable) until we see an alternative path worth treading. Some of us find it difficult to resist the allure of extreme grief emotion and its immobilizing effects. Some are less flexible or adaptable than others, flourishing in a more limited range of experience and activity; some are better able than others to imagine alternative courses of action, discern which alternative is best for us, and find motivation for action. Some are plagued by fear and anxiety about the uncertain future. Some are more comfortably autonomous than others. Finally, some incline more than others to use less effective coping strategies, sustaining denial or refusing to acknowledge the death itself and its impacts on our lives, determinedly avoiding the tasks at hand through diversion or keeping busy, or living exclusively in the present moment while refusing either to come to terms with the painful past or to face an all too frightening future.

Bill and Diane are young and healthy adults, whereas Margaret is older and more physically fragile. Bill, always physically vigorous, invests great energy, even frenetic energy, in keeping busy. He is oblivious to the energy he expends, and his neglect of eating could lead to trouble. Fortunately, pounding his head did no damage, although it might have. Diane, less physically vigorous, inclines less toward great expenditure of energy in coping. Her lethargy and her perceptible fragility may derive from growing physical exhaustion. Margaret's agitation and chronic sleeplessness threaten serious physical consequences and complicate her coping.

Like Bill, Diane, and Margaret, we are all subject to limitations or our ability to cope *physically*. As we address the innumerable tasks of grieving, the required effort saps our energy and drains our endurance and stamina. The more extensive the array of tasks we face, the more likely our grieving is to become an enervating and exhausting ordeal. Some of us simply are better prepared than others for the physical challenges of dealing with loss. The physically fragile, the ill, and the physically disabled are at greater risk for physical complication in their grieving. Moreover, some of us neglect our physical needs for rest, food, shelter, or treatment of physical ailments, in times of crisis. Failure to maintain good health and to attend to physical needs can compromise all other facets of our coping.

Neither Bill nor Diane can provide the full social support the other needs, despite their great mutual concern. Neither wishes to add demands to the nearly overwhelming burdens facing the other. Each is grateful for the other's continuing presence and sustained gentleness, patience, and affection. Bill's proud independence and his private nature make him uncomfortable in reaching out to all but those closest to him. Self-disclosure is very painful for him. When he does open up to a family member or friend, he is inarticulate about just what troubles him. He doubts the competence of mental health professionals, but he thinks of approaching his minister. Diane more readily reaches out to others. She tells her story adeptly and effectively solicits helping responses that she readily accepts. She finds the support group especially helpful as it provides a time and place for her to be with others who are not disturbed by her pain and who empathize because they have had similar experiences.

Margaret reaches out to Earl, who blocks her attempt to seek his support. She avoids Bill and Diane because she knows they suffer terribly. Because she does not want to burden her children with her problems, she neither reaches out to her other surviving children nor accepts their offers to help. She is proudly independent and stubbornly believes that people should take care of themselves. She is consequently reluctant to seek the professional support she almost certainly requires to deal with the trauma that so inhibits and complicates her normal grieving. She may call her minister.

Like Bill, Diane, and Margaret, we are also vulnerable to our limited capacities to cope *socially*.[14] Some of us more than others sense that we need the support of others. Sometimes we are blind to our own needs for social support or to the potential comfort, consolation, and support that others can provide. Some of us are inhibited in reaching out for support by pride in our independence, reluctance to burden others, unwillingness to take the initiative, inability to signal our needs, shyness, fear of admitting or showing vulnerability, anxiety about losing control of emotion, fear of rejection or insensitivity, or anxiety that others will retreat because they do not know what to do or say. Some mourners who do reach out to others are able to communicate just what troubles them or identify what response would help most. Some decline to accept support when it is offered. Sometimes mourners put off caregivers as they become too demanding, volatile, complaining, or ungrateful. Some hold views that only certain persons should provide support, for example, close family members or friends, and neither seek nor accept support from others, such as clergy, mental health professionals or support groups.

Bill, Diane, and Margaret only gradually grasp the nearly pervasive impacts of their losses on virtually every dimension of their being and every aspect of their lives. The enormity of their losses boggles their minds as they see how much they had taken for granted. Because Bill lives straightforwardly and is less self-aware or self-reflective, what he doesn't understand about himself and what happens to him confuses and frightens him. Diane, more self-aware and self-reflective, is less confused. Still, the devastation in her life frightens her. Margaret, so caught in the horror of what she has seen, barely notices the "ordinary" transformations in herself and her life pattern. All three think of grieving as something that happens to them, and none clearly perceives the range of tasks to be addressed. This thought of grief to be endured compounds their feelings of helplessness. Having taken every precaution imaginable to protect his family, Bill more than the others fixes on how the gas leak occurred.

The losses raise spiritual concerns. All three question why children suffer and die and wonder about the meanings of their children's abbreviated lives. They had believed that the just prosper, hard work and devotion to family bring great rewards, and bad things do not happen to good people. The deaths have loosened these cornerstones of their self-definition and family life. Bill stops going to church and considers leaving the church altogether, but life without it frightens him. He thinks he may one day approach his minister. Diane takes vague comfort in her continued affiliation with the church but approaches her minister for understanding of how what happened to her and her children is compatible with teachings around which she built her life. Spiritual questions plague both Bill and Diane as they wonder about the wisdom of starting a new family. Margaret clings to her faith and draws consolation from the sustaining belief that she will be reunited one day with her daughter and grandchildren.

None is at peace with what has happened. All three struggle to hope again and to sense that life has meaning and purpose. Bill and Diane, as they plan a new family and establish a new home, seem resilient and filled with hope, but they wonder whether they are being driven by desperation. They doubt that their lives will ever be as meaningful or purposeful as they once were. Margaret is not as hopeful and wonders whether she can live meaningfully again, given the devastation her nightmares bring.

Like Bill, Diane, and Margaret, we are vulnerable in our *intellectual and spiritual* limitations. Some of us more readily than others find comprehensible and satisfactory answers to questions about the causes of illness, accident, and death. Some of us better understand what happens to us in bereavement. Limits of self-awareness and self-reflection determine the extent of our surprise at how much of life we took for granted, our vagueness about what troubles us, our fright and apprehension, and our confusion and disorientation as we address the tasks of grieving. Some of us better understand the grieving process itself and are clearer about the challenges before us. Some more ably find (or retain) meaningful answers to abstract questions such as "Why is there death and suffering?," "Why must children die?," and "What are the meanings of life, death and suffering?" Some of us better tolerate living without answers to such questions. Some more easily avoid hopelessness, despair, purposelessness, and meaninglessness. Some of us are more resilient and more easily find peace and consolation. Some more readily discern and reaffirm what is left of meaningful connections previously established. Some of us more easily establish new ones.

Bill's truncated grieving of his sister Kim's death affects his ability to cope with his children's deaths. Kim died when Bill was a teenager seeking his own identity. He was inhibited about expressing his distress and his needs and did not receive adequate support from his peers. That experience set a troubling precedent for him, and his present losses tear through his well-built defenses. Diane reached her late twenties without ever having experienced major loss. She is utterly unprepared for the multiple loss of her children and her sister. Many of Margaret's peers and near-peers have died, and she is resigned to more of the same. However, she invests great hope in the generations coming after, and the losses of a child and her grandchildren profoundly upset her expectations. Parents and grandparents simply should not have to endure such losses, she believes.

Like Bill, Diane, and Margaret, we are also vulnerable to limitations in our coping capacities deriving from our *personal histories with loss*. Past loss and grieving shadow our present bereavement. Some of us have failed to grieve past losses effectively. Some have buried or inhibited our own grieving process or developed ineffective grieving patterns. Some of us are in the midst of unresolved grieving when another loss occurs. The ways we have coped previously tend to set precedents for our present coping. Few of us break with unhappy precedents in the ways we cope without self-conscious effort or guidance and encouragement from others. Some of us are already intensely grieving other recent losses when new bereavement compounds the impacts and challenges and takes us beyond our capacity to cope effectively. Some of us simply lack experience with grieving; the unprecedented experience surprises and catches us unprepared to deal with challenges that we perceive to be unlike any we've faced before.

Children are especially vulnerable, because they lack developed coping capacities. Unprecedented feelings frighten some and leave them at a loss as to what to do or say. Some imagine wrongly that they are responsible for the death, for example, because they wished the person dead. Loss often disrupts or undermines the development of self-confidence, self-esteem, and identity. Some feel helpless and need to learn that they have choices in response to choiceless events. Regressive behavior is common, as is reenactment in play. Children lack models for, and need guidance and support in finding, appropriate things to do in the mourning period and in putting together new life patterns. Dependence often makes them more anxious about the basic necessities of life, including food, shelter, and love. Death often breaks bonds just when children are testing and learning to value and trust them. The myth that children do not grieve leads some of us to neglect them and to exclude them from family or community responses to death. Some children lack the verbal ability to explain what troubles them, express their thoughts, feelings, and other reactions, or state what they need or hope for in response. Bereaved children confront many new questions and lack the support that settled answers provide. Their reality changes, too, but because they lack a developed orientation to reality prior to the death, they face greater disorientation unless someone answers their questions honestly and helps them understand what the realities of death and loss entail. What they overhear or misunderstand in adult conversation often confuses them. They typically lack mature beliefs about such things as the meanings of life, death, and suffering. Some realize for the first time that they, too, could die, especially if the deceased was a sibling or a peer. Similarly, the retarded or demented are especially vulnerable in their undeveloped or diminished coping capacities. And some otherwise mature adults simply lack maturity in some facet of personal development and are consequently less prepared to cope.

We Are Vulnerable in Challenging Social Circumstances

Bill's family has coped with previous loss through avoidance. His own family supports him little, and he is uncomfortable both in Diane's family and in the support group. His best friend, Diane, is clearly caught up in her own grief and unable to offer the support and comfort he needs. His other friends do not know what to do or say to comfort or console him. Diane is fortunate in the support provided by her surviving brothers and sisters, but still she reaches out to the parents' support group. While she fully understands their current limitations, she nevertheless misses the support of those who usually helped most: her best friend, Bill, her sister, Mary, and her mother, Margaret. Her father, Earl, is inaccessible, but he always has been. Earl's lack of emotional support dismays Margaret, but she resigns herself to its inadequacy. His expectation that she can somehow manage to keep her mind on other things is simply unrealistic for her, and it strikes her as nearly cruel. Charitably, she suspects he is simply unable to deal with any admixture of her pain with his.

Like Bill, Diane, and Margaret, we grieve not in isolation but in social contexts where we live with family and friends and within cultural settings and surrounding communities. In interaction with family and peers we develop our identities, take on roles, accumulate histories with loss, and see others as models for dealing with loss. Some of us bring to present grieving histories of inadequate support and poor modeling. Some of us are troubled as others bring unwelcome expectations to bear on us. Some of us are estranged, alienated, or otherwise socially distant from those from whom we most need support. Some around us are themselves bereaved and unable to provide the support we need.

Bill and Diane both take little comfort in traditional beliefs and hesitate to express doubts about them to their minister. Bill resents the too glib dismissal of his grief at the Rotary Club, envies Diane's openness, and perhaps wonders about the fairness of society's expectations about men who grieve. What, exactly, does it mean to "be strong" in such times of need? Diane takes comfort in the support provided a grieving mother but hurts to see Bill having such difficulty in finding and accepting support. Margaret recognizes that Earl simply knows no other way but resents the culture that made him what he is. She feels confined in her role as wife and mother.

Our cultural heritage, too, helps define how we will react to loss in behavior, emotion, and understanding. For some of us this cultural influence interferes in or inhibits our grieving. Some of us find traditional mourning practices unhelpful or experience cultural norms and social rules as confining and inflexible. Some of us find traditional beliefs unsupportive or inadequate; some resent the intolerance of others or their lack of sympathy for spiritual questioning and crisis. Some of us are troubled by cultural expectations that we no longer accept, including expectations associated with such things as religion, family, gender, or age.

As we participate in, for example, the world of work, a church, or the broader social community, we become vulnerable to unrealistic demands made on us by virtue of our having taken on those affiliations. Some of us are torn between a desire to be in society and a desire to retreat from it. Some of us feel out of rhythm with daily living in society, fail to fulfill our functions, and suffer censure. Bill is his own boss and returns to work to keep busy, not out of financial necessity or perceived risk of offending his boss or losing his job. Bill and Diane are torn between retreat from community involvement for a time and a desire to continue to contribute.

We are vulnerable to abuses of power and authority, for example, from a controlling head of family, a manipulative life's companion, an unreasonable boss, or a paternalistic social service or health-care provider. Children, and others in subordinate positions because of their perceived or real lack of maturity, are especially vulnerable to power plays that deny them the opportunity to grieve at all or to grieve on their own terms. When we trust professional caregivers, we are especially vulnerable to inappropriate caregiver control of our experiences, no matter how well intentioned. Fortunately, such abuses of power have had no place in Bill's, Diane's, or Margaret's experience, although Margaret struggles to resist that interpretation of Earl's behavior.

Finally, misunderstanding and bad advice and counsel about grief abound, and some among us accept such advice and allow it to distort our self-understanding and our way of coping with loss. For some of us, support from social service and mental health agencies, religious organizations, and support groups is inadequate, unavailable, or inaccessible. Disenfranchisement compounds our grief when we perceive that social support would be available were it not for the stigmatized character of our relationship with the deceased.

Respecting Loss in Others

Having others understand us as we flourish and in our vulnerability is not sufficient to ensure respect for our individuality. Yes, respect for us as we grieve requires that those who care about and for us understand how we have flourished in meaningful and purposeful experiences, actions, and connections within our own individual life patterns prior to our bereavement. Respect also requires that they understand how we are vulnerable both to the disruption of life patterns that bereavement entails and to factors that compromise, hinder, interfere with, or undermine our ability to cope effectively. Like Bill, Diane, and Margaret, we must be known in our distinctive ways of flourishing and in our particular vulnerabilities and limitations.

Respect also requires that these understandings shape others' interactions with us. At the least, respect requires that caregivers avoid exacerbating our vulnerability or interfering with us as we cope in our own ways. To fail to do so undercuts our autonomy as we give direction to our own lives and seek again to flourish and find daily purpose and meaning in life,[15] it also compounds our deprivation, delays progress in our grieving, and postpones our returning to flourishing in viable, reestablished life patterns. Full respect requires more, however, than this minimal restraint from interference in our coping. It requires actions that acknowledge and promote community with us and thereby contribute to our return to flourishing.[16] Noninterference in our lives does not suffice to sustain community with us, because loss severely compromises our capacities to flourish and to find purpose and meaning in life. These capacities can be sustained in most cases only through maintenance of bonds with, and active support from, those around us. Grieving revives both our appreciation of the possibility for continued purpose and meaning and our motivation to resume involvement in daily life and to find new direction in our life stories despite our losses. Constructive support and active helping preserve our community membership, facilitate our grieving, enable our return to flourishing, and contribute to our reestablishing viable life patterns.

As we care about and for those among us who are grieving, respect for their individuality requires that we recognize the potentially far-reaching impacts of loss on their lives. We can actively and constructively support their individual struggles by letting them know that we understand that grieving takes much time and energy. We can offer patience, flexibility, and forgiveness in our expectations of them at home, at work, and in other roles and relationships. We can encourage them to seek advice and support from the sources they think will be most helpful. We can offer our own presence and reassure them that our affection, care, concern, and empathy will remain constant. We can make ourselves available to listen actively, offer constructive advice when we are asked, and provide comfort and support as requested. We can acknowledge the legitimacy of their grieving and discourage others from disenfranchising or abandoning them at a time when they most need community support. We can help the bereaved to understand grieving as an active coping process, encourage them to resist passivity and helplessness, and reinforce and support their self-confidence and self-esteem. We can encourage them to engage actively in grieving at their own pace and in their own ways. We can attune ourselves to the distinctive contours of their experiences and recognize and respond sensitively to the points of their greatest vulnerability. We can support and encourage them as they exercise their well-developed coping skills, address their unique tasks, and define their own path to renewed flourishing. Where their coping abilities are limited, we should avoid paternalism, help them to learn how to be more autonomous, support and encourage them as they develop new coping skills, and motivate them to think of desirable outcomes of their grieving as outlined in Chapter 2. In these ways we can demonstrate respect for their individuality even as we affirm community with them.

What Our Self-Respect Requires

Bill postpones decisions he is not yet ready to make about some items in his home. He gives himself time to conclude that he cannot return to live in the house where his children and Mary died. He dismisses the poor advice of his friends at Rotary. He recognizes his own discomfort in the support group and with Diane's family, even as he acknowledges the value of the self-disclosure that is so difficult for him. He sees that the dispositions and behaviors of his sixteen-year-old self as he dealt with his sister Kim's death do not serve him well. And he begins to change that pattern as he returns to the children's graveside to cry privately. Should he become frustrated or stymied, he may feel and act on a need to reach out for the help of others, perhaps by returning to the support group with Diane or calling on his minister. Diane paces herself as she returns to sort through the house with Bill. She, too, recognizes that she cannot return to live there. She uses self-reflection and her expressive abilities to her advantage. Despite her tendency to defer to Bill, she seeks help independently. She recognizes that she needs the support of others and reaches out for and accepts it freely from her family and from the support group. Margaret has yet to muster the courage to defy Earl's controlling influence in her life and to reach out for the help that she sees she so desperately needs.

In all of these ways, Bill, Diane, and Margaret are struggling to maintain their own self-respect as they grieve. My notion of respect for individuality can be used to define a minimum of self-care that we owe ourselves when we grieve. Our self-respect requires that we understand how we can live with purpose and meaning and how we are vulnerable to the effects of bereavement, the limitations of our coping capacities, and the interferences of others as we grieve. Inattention to these matters adds to our suffering as it leaves our needs unrecognized and undermines our reestablishing meaningful life patterns. We owe it to ourselves actively to address the tasks of grieving out of respect for our own remaining potential to flourish again. We must acknowledge our vulnerability and avoid acting in ways that exacerbate it.

Bill lives very straightforwardly and is rarely self-reflective. Diane, in contrast, is far more introspective and self-aware. His self-respect does not require that Bill all of a sudden become much more like Diane. Bill grows painfully aware of how much he took for granted in life when his children were alive, but he need not dwell in that pain to be self-respecting. Indeed, the intensity of the pain tends to paralyze him. He copes more effectively and straightforwardly as he returns to his home and sorts what is left behind. Diane's pain at how much she took for granted motivates her to greater self-reflection. That reflection helps her more self-consciously to define ways of coping. Margaret, ordinarily instinctive and straightforward in coping with adversity, is stuck in the traumatic vision of the death scene.

These differences in Bill's, Diane's, and Margaret's coping make it clear that self-respect does not require that all of us become fully self-aware and self-reflective when we grieve. Self-respect does not require us to be utterly lucid about all we took for granted as we flourished in complex life patterns. Nor does it require that we be transparent to ourselves in our feelings, beliefs and ideas, habits and dispositions, motivations, and coping capacities. As individuals, we vary across a broad spectrum. At one end are those like Bill and Margaret, who live in a straight-ahead fashion with only marginal self-awareness and with self-reflection a rare occurrence. At the other end are those like Diane, who live in near-constant self-awareness and who are self-reflective at almost every turn. Self-respect is possible anywhere along this spectrum. To be sure, losses do stimulate self-awareness and self-reflection; most of us become more aware than ever, often painfully so, of the many elements of our life patterns that we have taken for granted. Still, self-respect does not require that we sustain whatever heightened self-awareness comes over us. Self-respect does not require that we abandon straight-ahead, non–self-reflective life patterns when grieving in that manner is effective for us.

Self-respect does require a minimal self-awareness (however visceral and inarticulate it may be) that allows us to recognize honestly when we have difficulty in meeting the challenges of grieving. We must not shrink from acknowledging our frustrations when we feel stuck or stymied. We must discern what dispositions lead us to such frustration, sense what it is about particular situations that triggers our dispositions, and understand how we act in ways that bring us into situations where we are frustrated or out of our depth. We must then adjust our dispositions and behaviors (as Bill does in going to the cemetery to cry privately) so that we do not continually frustrate ourselves and undermine our own grieving. Self-respect requires that we appreciate anew our existing strengths and capacities and use them to meet the challenges of grieving in order to flourish once again. Self-respect requries that we recognize when the interference of others frustrates our coping (as Earl's does Margaret's) and avoid or resist the interference. Finally, self-respect requires that we seek the respectful help and support of others when we sense that we have reached the limits of our coping capacities.[17]

Notes

1. See Victor Frankl, *Man's Search for Meaning: An Introduction to Logotherapy*, 3d ed. (New York: Touchstone Books, 1984).

2. Frankl, *Man's Search*.

3. See Robert Lifton, *The Broken Connection: On Death and the Continuity of Life* (New York: Basic Books, 1983), for a detailed treatment of the theme of the relation of experiences of connectedness and experienced meaningfulness in living.

4. The vulnerability of the bereaved to having to restructure their lives is treated more extensively in Chapter 5.

5. Complications in relationships with fellow survivors are treated separately later in this chapter.

6. See Therese Rando, *Treatment of Complicated Mourning* (Champaign, Ill.: Research Press, 1993), for extensive treatment of the topic of complicated grief in its many varieties.

7. See Chapter 4 for a fuller elaboration of the story of Ed's tragic loss of Bobby.

8. See Chapter 2 for detailed discussion of this emotion.

9. Doka, Kenneth, ed., *Disenfranchised Grief: Recognizing Hidden Sorrow* (Lexington, Mass.: Lexington Press, 1989).

10. Recall the story of Jennifer's near disenfranchisement in Chapter 2.

11. See Chapter 6 for elaboration of the story of Colleen's coming to terms with the suicide of her daughter Sheila.

12. Again, see Rando, *Complicated Mourning*.

13. See Chapter 2 for discussion of this emotion.

14. Here the focus is upon the limitations in social skills of the bereaved not the shortcomings of others' attempts to support them. The latter are treated more extensively later in this chapter.

15. In its second version, Kant's Categorical Imperative states that respect requires persons to "act so as to treat humanity, whether in your own person or in that of another, always as an end and never as a means only." Immanuel Kant, *Foundation of the Metaphysics of Morals*, trans. L. W. Beck in *Critique of Practical Reason and Other Writings in Moral Philosophy* (Chicago: University of Chicago Press, 1949).

16. In its third version, Kant's Categorical Imperative states that respect requires persons to "act according to the maxims of a universally legislative member of a merely potential kingdom of ends." Kant, *Foundation*.

17. It is interesting to consider the implications of the notion of self-respect for children and others whose coping capacities either are not fully developed or have been seriously and perhaps permanently diminished. Fuller treatment of this subject will have to wait for another occasion. It would include consideration of such things as a) the lack of fully developed notions of the separateness of persons or individual self-identity and b) what respect for persons requires in interaction with children and others who lack the capacity for self-respect.

4

Relearning the World

INTERREGNUM

The span between life and death
Can be as quick and sudden
As a puff of wind
That blows out a candle.
But the candle does not suffer
After darkness comes.
It is the person
Left in the dark room
Who gropes and stumbles.
                    Helen Duke Fike

At first I was very afraid of going to places where H.
and I had been happy—our favorite pub, or favorite wood.
But I decided to do it at once—like sending a pilot
up again as soon as possible after he's had a crash.
Unexpectedly, it makes no difference. Her absence is no
more emphatic in those places than anywhere else. It's
not local at all. . . . The act of living is different all
through. Her absence is like the sky, spread over
everything.

                    C. S. Lewis

The Story of Ed and Elise

Ed's son Bobby, age six, dies unexpectedly in the emergency room of
a hospital. Ed had brought Bobby there along with Elise, the child's
mother, following an accident at home with a small pistol Ed had
bought to protect his family while he was away on business. When
Bobby slipped into his parents' bedroom while playing with his

    The general outline of the thinking developed in this chapter was first devel-
oped in my "Relearning the World: On the Phenomenology of Grieving," in *Journal
of the British Society for Phenomenology* (1990).

99

friend David, the boys discovered the gun in a drawer by the bed. The gun went off accidentally in Bobby's hand, wounding him in the abdomen. He was bleeding but conscious when Ed and Elise arrived at the hospital only a few blocks from their home. Emergency personnel took Bobby from them promptly and removed him to another room for intensive attention. The parents waited for what seemed like hours, though by the clock it was but forty minutes. Both longed to be with Bobby. They knew he needed them.

The physician who attended their child calls Ed and Elise to a conference room. She assures them that although everything that could be done was done, Bobby died. She says that she is sorry, she will gladly answer any questions, a police report must be filed, and she will call a chaplain if they wish.

Ed screams in protest at the whole scene while Elise weeps uncontrollably. Ed feels trapped in a whirlwind of emotion. He feels guilt about buying the gun. He remembers his in-laws' repeated warning that having the gun in the house was dangerous, and he dreads telling them how Bobby died. He fears that Elise blames him. His heart races, and he is extremely agitated. He feels as if he had been punched in the stomach, and he gasps for breath. Beyond the first few words spoken by the doctor, he understands nothing. His surroundings recede into a hazy mist. Although he sees Elise's anguish, he feels too disconcerted to reach out to her. He needs comfort so desperately himself. Elise's silence is penetrating.

Elise feels helpless and overwhelmed. Events unfold at a pace that her coping capacities cannot match. Her surroundings recede as she senses herself withdrawing behind a curtain of unreality. Her intense weeping frightens her. She feels guilty for not protesting along with her parents when Ed bought the gun. She feels that she failed to protect her son. She hears Ed's screams, and her ambivalence toward him renders her silent. She feels inconsolable and lost.

Ed questions the doctor about whether he and Elise were right to bring Bobby themselves rather than wait for an ambulance. He cannot tell whether the doctor offers reassurance sincerely or merely as a gesture of consolation. His mind fills with more questions than he can voice: "How can this be?" and "Why did this have to happen?" He dreads speaking to the police about the accident. "Can't they leave good people alone at times like these?" he thinks. The doctor notices Ed's agitation and Elise's pain and offers tranquilizers. Both refuse, recognizing that they are not fully lucid as it is and not wanting to miss what each senses is a pivotal experience.

Ed insists that he and Elise be allowed to see Bobby. He wants to confirm what he cannot take in without seeing for himself. The visit is emotionally excruciating. He, like Elise, weeps uncontrollably when he sees and holds the lifeless body of the child who hours before had been playing innocently before them. Yet both welcome the opportunity, through their tears, to again be with Bobby, say private good-byes, and thank him for having touched their lives in so many ways.

Through her tears, Elise asks to meet with the chaplain. He joins them in the room with Bobby. The chaplain assures them that over time the meaning of the events of the day will become clearer and the pain will subside. The assurances provide little comfort, and Ed and Elise resist believing them. Questions burn within them both, questions they hold within because neither expects the seemingly too facile chaplain to answer usefully: "Is this some kind of punishment from God or a terrible random happening?" "Why is there suffering and death?" "Why must little children die?" "What kind of world is this where such promising life can be cut short?" "Why did Bobby live?" Ed feels abandoned by God in his hour of need, and Elise feels victimized and cheated by terrible events beyond her control. They feel helpless, hopeless, and alone in sorrow.

David has been nearly forgotten in the rush of events to bring Bobby for medical attention. Fortunately, he lives next door, and Elise had brought him home to his mother's arms as Ed brought Bobby to the car to go to the hospital. Elise did not explain and David's mother knew little of what happened. David is stunned. He says nothing not only because of the shock but also because he lacks the words to express what he is experiencing. The event shatters the innocence of his world. His mother sees this, despairs of being able to help him for the long term, but offers the comfort of her warm, sheltering arms as she awaits further news of Bobby.

The chaplain urges that the other children at home, Bobby's older brother and sister, Johnny and Melanie, need their parents' attention. He encourages the couple to return home to them. Ed and Elise dread the return home. When they arrive, Ed listens, speechless, as Elise tells Johnny and Melanie the awful news. Each is stunned. Johnny, sixteen, runs out the front door in angry silence. Melanie, eleven, weeps and hugs her mother. Elise welcomes the hug but takes no comfort in it. Again, Ed feels helpless and alone. Only later that evening does Elise call to tell David's mother that Bobby has died.

The funeral seems but a necessary formality. A minister attempts to offer peace and consolation through words that Ed and Elise hear as but a string of meaningless clichés and platitudes. Ed and Elise remember little other than the fact that so many mourners attend. Many lavish attention on Elise. Ed longs for warm embraces, not firm handshakes. Many friends volunteer to help later; none follow through.

After the funeral, Ed and Elise return home. Bobby's death haunts Ed in every corner of his home. Ed's own bedroom is now a death chamber, and he sleeps in the den. He closes the door to Bobby's room, resolved to deal with its contents some other time, he knows not when. Still, he confronts with mixed feelings the early drawings and paintings on that door and on the refrigerator. He hurts when he sees them, feels close to Bobby, and senses that Elise wants them to remain in place lest they sever still more ties to him. Ed moves Bobby's toys, scattered in the family room and elsewhere, into Bobby's room. He clusters the toys in the garage in a corner and covers them with a blanket. No matter where he eats, he notices that Bobby's place is no longer occupied. The swing set in the backyard is too well anchored in cement to allow for easy removal, so he avoids either entering the yard or looking toward it through the family room window. It seems to him there is no place in his home where he can escape Bobby's memory. It is not that he wants to forget Bobby, but for now it is often terrible to remember. The lack of respite nearly overwhelms him. He begins to wonder whether it is realistic to expect to stay in the house. He hesitates to voice his concern for fear of further upsetting and disrupting the lives of his family.

The return to work affords none of the distraction Ed thinks he needs. First, he sees the toy corner in the garage. Then, he recalls how Bobby so often sat beside him while he drove, studying carefully how he did it, asking questions about the controls, chattering ceaselessly, and looking excitedly at places along the way. He changes his route to avoid David's house and Bobby's school and favorite playground. On arrival at work, he confronts the family photos on his desk. He feels as if putting them away would be like putting Bobby away, so he relocates them in order to avoid seeing Bobby's face as often during the day. He continues to use the coffee mug that Bobby gave him for his birthday, sometimes weeping as he does and sometimes daydreaming.

It is difficult for Ed to find refuge from his pain. He is reminded of Bobby wherever he turns. He walks alone in the evenings to escape the tensions at home. But he senses Bobby's absence everywhere he goes: in the neighborhood where Bobby and he walked or rode bicycles together or where Bobby's friends and schoolmates live; in the parks where the family played together and enjoyed picnics; or downtown where he bought things for Bobby, helped Bobby select Christmas and birthday gifts for others, stopped for a pizza, ice cream, cookies, or family dinner, took in a movie, or played games in the arcade. He goes to Bobby's grave often, talks with him there, seeks his forgiveness, and simply feels close. He cannot bring himself to return to church. He knows it is supposed to be a place where he can find comfort, consolation, and even forgiveness. However, he expects that the reminder of Bobby sitting next to him there would be too painful. He does not wish to allow himself to be at peace with what he feels he has done. As he feels abandoned, he longs for God to know him in his anguish. He feels not ready for God's forgiveness when he cannot forgive himself.

Ed cannot grasp just why or where he fits in. He is not of phase with his daily routine. The death, the life now ended, and the emptiness pervade every waking hour. He desperately needs comfort; he does not find it. Interactions with friends and coworkers often irritate him. He feels responsible for Johnny and Melanie's grief but is unable to reach out to help them. He fears that the lingering tensions with Elise will bring an end to his marriage and add further chaos to his life. Though Elise joins a support group for bereaved parents, he is reluctant to go with her for fear of the exposure. There seems no end to the pain. He is drained. There is no prospect of relief. It seems to him that the world has gone mad. His hopes barely extend beyond the next hours to the next day, and his future seems bleak. He sees the same in Elise, knows she needs him, and feels impotent to help.

Elise, too, notices Bobby's absence wherever she turns. He is too much with her in the home that seems at once filled with memories yet hauntingly empty. She, too, chooses to sleep in a different room to avoid the bedroom where he died. Sometimes, when Ed and the children are gone, she enters Bobby's room, sits on his bed, looks around the room, and screams or weeps. She stays until she can stand it no longer. She senses that Ed would like the drawings on Bobby's door removed and is glad he says nothing because she fears she would explode if forced to take them down. She is relieved that Ed has removed the toys to Bobby's room. She can see them when she wants, and she and Ed can decide what to do with them later. Each room holds special memories. At first, the memories are painful, but gradually she begins to find comfort in knowing that she at least has them. Yet, she, too, wonders whether the house can ever again feel like home. She hesitates to say anything to Ed for fear of adding to his obvious guilt.

Elise at times envies Ed the escape she imagines he finds in going to work. She has little idea of how often Ed is reminded of Bobby while on the way to and on the job. Her daily labors are at home. She approaches the work halfheartedly, and she cuts back considerably in her daily efforts. She feels she must do the bare minimum to maintain a semblance of order and to provide Johnny and Melanie with what they need. While in the kitchen, she does her best to avert her eyes from the window view of David's house. When she finds the energy to clean, she constantly revisits experiences with Bobby in every room. Her anger mounts when she nears the bedroom where Bobby was both conceived and shot. Other rooms are filled with happy memories, and she especially likes to retreat to the family room for tea and quiet reflection. She often pauses before the drawings on Bobby's door and the refrigerator, and she sometimes takes a favorite portrait from the wall and holds it close to her heart.

Elise, too, finds little refuge from her pain. She hasn't the energy to walk in the evenings with Ed and can't understand how he finds any comfort in passing so many places that must remind him of Bobby. Her daily routine takes her to stores and malls often and to Melanie's school, where Bobby had just begun first grade. Even places where she only occasionally had taken Bobby prove problematic as clerks and other workers ask about her little boy, not realizing that he has died. She is grateful for solitude whenever she can find it. She dreads going to her parents' home where Bobby so enjoyed playing and where she fears her parents will not remain silent about the gun. She sometimes goes to Bobby's grave during the day, talks with him there, meditates or prays, and senses that he knows she is there. She attends church alone but understands Ed's reluctance to join her. Again, she senses that Bobby is close in church and that he is in good hands. This comforts and consoles her and leads her to begin to recognize how much Ed needs her forgiveness as well as Bobby's, God's, and, ultimately, his own. She prays for help in understanding how to forgive Ed and how her son's death is compatible with God's goodness. She prays for a return of the contentment and safety in God's arms she once knew.

Elise sees little point in daily routine as the loss preoccupies her. She is lethargic, unable to concentrate or find meaning in any activity. She struggles to revive hopes and aspirations for her family's future, but she doubts she will ever find life as meaningful again in a world that seems so much more threatening and arbitrary than before. Friends and family seem unable to do or say anything that comforts her. She joins a support group and finds great relief as she learns that others have experienced similar losses and at least begun to deal with the turmoil it introduced into their lives. She hopes eventually to draw Ed into going with her. Her daily efforts on Johnny's and Melanie's behalf and her interactions with them remind her that she now has only two living children and leave her feeling inadequate to attend to their needs as children whose little brother has died. She is exhausted. She knows Ed feels terrible, but she does not know how to approach him. She fears that if she does not find a way to forgive him, she will lose her marriage as well.

Ed and Elise, and many who suffer terrible losses, would have little trouble identifying with Alfred Lord Tennyson when he wrote:

> Dark house, by which once more I stand
>   Here in the unlovely street,
>   Doors, where my heart was used to beat
> So quickly, waiting for a hand,
>
> A hand that can be clasped no more—
>   Behold me, for I cannot sleep,
>   And like a guilty thing I creep
> At earliest morning to the door.
>
> He is not here, but far away
>   The noise of life begins again,
>   And ghastly thro' the drizzling rain
> On the bald street breaks the blank day.[1]

How We Relearn Our Worlds

When Ed and Elise return home first from the hospital where Bobby has died and later from Bobby's funeral and burial, they face a world that is changed utterly by what has happened. They can never experience, or be at home in, that world in the same way they were prior to Bobby's death. They are reminded of Bobby's absence everywhere, by the things he has left behind, in the places where they shared life with him, in interaction with one another and with others who survive with them, and in their own minds and hearts where they came to know and love him. Relearning their worlds is not simply a matter of registering Bobby's absence or taking in new information about the world as it is now without him. It is a struggle to discover, and make their own, ways of going on without him in that world. So much of what they had taken for granted in their lives is no longer sustainable, at least not in the way it was prior to Bobby's death. The story of their grieving is the story of finding new places for themselves, shaping new daily routines, establishing new patterns of experience, achievement, and connection, and giving new direction to their life stories in the particular contexts of their lives. In each of these broad struggles the relearning engages them as whole persons, in all facets of their being. How, if they choose to, will each carry on in their home where they raised Bobby, laughed and cried with him, and where they found him after he fatally wounded himself? What will it be like for each of them to deal with the things that Bobby has left behind or once again to be in places they had been with him? How, if at all, will each be a friend, companion, or lover for the other, given their beliefs about responsibility for what happened? How are they to be parents to Johnny and Melanie, who are themselves now Bobby's bereaved brother and sister? How will they face and interact with neighbors and with David's parents, given what David has witnessed? How will each come to terms with Elise's parents, who had warned Ed not to buy the gun? How, if at all, will they find ways of saying good-bye to Bobby while retaining love for him in their lives? How is each to come again to feel at home in the greater scheme of things, at peace with God? What can each do or say to begin to introduce order into the chaos of their lives? What will motivate them as they reshape their daily routines at home, at work, in interaction with others? How will each recover a sense of daily purpose? What will ground hope for the future for each and a sense that life is meaningful?

Like Ed and Elise, each of us is the subject of an ongoing experience of the world with a unique contour and integrity worthy of respect. Loss of another through death affects, often profoundly, the entire fabric of our experiencing and acting in the world. Bereavement challenges us to relearn virtually all components of our worlds as we experience them.[2] As it does for Ed and Elise, losses transform the world as we experience it, sometimes pervasively. Coming to terms with the changes requires that we relearn the world. Before we consider the extent of what we may have to relearn, let us consider the nature of the relearning itself.[3]

As we, like Ed and Elise, find our ways in the world (that is, learn it in the first place), we do not simply master information and develop theoretical constructs to organize and systematize that information. Rather, we experience the world in fundamentally practical terms before we attempt to reflect or theorize about it or our experience. We live life, for the most part, straightforwardly, not self-reflectively. We discern the value and significance of what we encounter in the light of our acquired and often cherished goals, hopes, and aspirations. We sometimes realize, and at other times seek, find, and appropriate, meanings in what we experience. We find our bearings in the world and give direction to, and seek a sense of purpose in, our ongoing living. So, too, finding our way in the world after bereavement, that is, relearning the world, is not a matter of *learning information about the world* but *learning how to be and act in the world* differently in the light of our loss.

As we live, we establish, broaden, enrich, combine, transform, and at times discard or abandon practical involvements with things, places, other persons, and projects. We develop and achieve individual character through our patterns of caring and through the variety, breadth, and depth of our attachments to the surrounding world. Our life histories unfold as we weave and reweave these threads of attachment. Bereavement rends, and sometimes threatens to completely unravel, the fabric of our caring involvement in the world; as we grieve, we struggle to reweave the fabric and establish a new integrity in our pattern of caring involvement.

As we establish life patterns, we come to take much for granted. We experience such aspects of our lives as given, settled, unquestioned; only rarely are they the object of reflection. Rather, the taken-for-granted aspects of our lives take shape and operate anonymously, habitually, and automatically as working assumptions in daily living.[4] These assumptions provide us with well-established interpretations of the world; they orient us within the world and function as the basis for our interaction with the diverse elements that make up that world.

We do not take for granted only cognitive assumptions as we engage in the world. We also take for granted the emotional and psychological, behavioral, physical and biological, social, and spiritual aspects of our experience and activity. We experience the pain of the emotion grief when we bring dispositions to feel, behave, think, expect, and hope as if the deceased still lived to a world where he or she no longer lives.[5] Relearning the world is a multifaceted transitional process. As we grieve, we appropriate new understandings of the world and ourselves within it. We also become different in the light of the loss as we assume a new orientation to the world. As we relearn, we adjust emotional and other psychological responses and postures. We transform habits, motivations, and behaviors. We find new ways to meet biological needs. We reshape our interactions and connections with others. And we change understandings and interpretations and alter spiritual perspectives. Relearning is thus holistic. Our grieving is organic, and we experience it organically. These facets of grieving interweave intimately as we grieve.

As we relearn the world, we make two kinds of accommodations in relation to what we took for granted prior to the death. Some of what we took for granted in ourselves or in our life patterns is no longer viable or sustainable. Relearning the world thus requires that we make changes, more or less self-consciously. Some of what we took for granted in ourselves or in our life patterns, however, does remain viable. The death (in itself an event we perhaps assumed would not happen, at least not then) may shake us so much that we hestitate to trust even what does remain viable in our life patterns. Relearning the world thus requires that we identify, test, and recover trust in what remains viable, rather than define and appropriate new ways of being in the world.

The Worlds We Relearn

We experience the world (and must relearn it as we grieve) as the encompassing context of our cares and concerns. We experience the world prior to any reflection as the place where we engage in activities and undertake projects. We experience ourselves as more or less at home in the world in our everyday lives and undertakings and in the broader scheme of things. We experience the world as filled with objects we care about and with supports for or hindrances to our projects. Three major spheres of such care and concern together constitute the world we must relearn in grieving. We experience the objects, places, natural contexts, and conditions in our physical environment as useful or as having other significance for our projects and the meanings of our lives. We experience others in our families and broader communities as either objects of care and concern in their own right or as persons with whom we share the world and whose presence influences the pattern of our care and concern. We experience ourselves as we understand our own identities (in terms of, for example, our personal histories, present commitments, hopes and aspirations, and convictions), take responsibility for our decisions and projects more or less self-confidently, and think well or ill of ourselves. Within each of these broad spheres, when we grieve we meet definable types of challenges, address tasks, and make choices about appropriate and effective means of addressing those tasks and challenges. Ed and Elise must come to terms with objects and places and complications in relationships with fellow survivors. And they must learn who they are now, struggle with their shaken self-confidence, and reevaluate the worth of their own lives.

We Relearn Our Physical Surroundings

The most obvious element of our world is our physical surroundings. As Ed and Elise return home, they are painfully aware that their house cannot be the same home it was before the accident. After they continue to live in it for a time, each recognizes (but neither voices) the need to decide whether to stay in the house that so unsettles them. Their bedroom is now the scene of Bobby's fatal accident. Each decides independently and temporarily to sleep elsewhere. Later, they may decide to resume sleeping in the room, redecorate it first, change the use of the room and convert another room into a bedroom for the two of them, or leave the house for another because the room is filled with too many painful reminders. Each chooses to deal with Bobby's room differently. Ed keeps the door closed, avoids it, and, at least temporarily, postpones dealing with the pain he expects to feel when he reenters the room. Elise, in contrast, enters the room, screams, weeps, and stays until she can no longer stand it, all seemingly in an effort to work through the pain that being in the room arouses. Later, Ed and Elise may decide to enter the room together simply to experience it or to begin to sort its contents.

Each must also cope with places special and not so special within their home, for example, Bobby's favorite play areas, his places at the kitchen and the dining room tables, and places where he learned important lessons, shared good times, or was disciplined.

Outside the home Ed changes his route to work to avoid David's house, Bobby's school, and playgrounds. Yet he walks the neighborhood and the downtown area in the evenings and notices Bobby's absence in many places where he did not anticipate doing so. Elise returns to Bobby's school because Melanie still attends classes there and continues to shop where she had with Bobby. Later, she may choose to join Ed on his walks, or they may decide to move to an entirely different neighborhood. Elise hesitates to visit her parents' home to avoid any confrontation about the gun, but it is doubtful she will stay away indefinitely. Both Ed and Elise take comfort in visiting Bobby's grave, though for now they choose to go separately. Ed insisted that Bobby's casket be placed at the front of the church during the funeral, in part because the week before his son died, Ed had refused Bobby's plea to be allowed to sit in the front row.

Ed chooses for now not to return to church. Elise, by contrast, chooses to attend church regularly and finds comfort and consolation there. In the future Ed and Elise may or may not return to favorite vacations spots or go to places where they had only hoped to take Bobby. Each will almost certainly be reminded of Bobby's life and absence in unexpected places at inopportune times. Neither can anticipate every encounter with places that will prompt both new grieving and a reevaluation of their ways of caring about the physical world.

Similarly, Ed and Elise must learn to deal with the things in their lives. They have postponed sorting the contents of Bobby's room in part because packing things away or otherwise disposing of them seems equivalent to disposing of Bobby. For now, Ed has stashed items that were scattered around the house in Bobby's room or under the blanket in the garage to be dealt with later. If it is easy to decide to dispose of the toothbrush and other toilet articles, actually doing so may not be as easy. It will be far harder to decide what to do with the sweater Grandma made and the baseball glove Bobby was just learning to use. Eventually, Ed and Elise must deal with all that Bobby has left behind: personal effects, odd "little-boy stuff" hidden in drawers and shoe boxes in the closet, clothing, toys, drawings, paintings, hangings on the wall, remnants from his first efforts at school, and the swing set in the backyard. Each must reassess the meanings of the photos and other mementos on the walls and in the family albums. For now, they choose to leave his drawings and the family pictures in place (both at home and at Ed's office) though each reacts differently to them. They may choose to keep some things, give Johnny and Melanie opportunities to select items to help them remember Bobby, offer some things to nieces, nephews, or friends of their children, donate some to charitable organizations, throw some in the trash, or set some aside in the attic or garage for still later disposition. After the shooting, and prior to the funeral, the police came to the house for a routine investigation and confiscated the gun; when they inform Ed that they are ready to release the weapon, he must choose whether to tell Elise and decide with her what to do with it, accept it without saying anything to her, or dispose of it. Ed and Elise may experience different emotions in response to things of significance in Bobby's life, face them more or less reluctantly, differ about what to do with them, tolerate more or less well the other's being party to the decisions, or attach different meanings to them. Neither can anticipate every encounter with objects or places that will prompt both new grieving and a reevaluation of their ways of caring about the physical world.

Johnny and Melanie must also relearn their physical environments, including the home they shared with Bobby and the places they visited together, some probably unknown to either Ed or Elise. Objects and places arouse varied memories and emotional responses and have different meanings for each of them. Their parents may not be aware of the significance of particular objects or places for them. Moreover, Ed and Elise may decide to do things with or about objects or places that limit their children's options. Johnny and Melanie may choose to voice their concerns or preferences if these decisions bother them or to keep silent. For example, Ed and Elise may or may not include Johnny or Melanie in the decision about whether to stay in the house. If they choose to move, this may or may not affect where Johnny or Melanie attends school, how easy it is to visit friends, and other aspects of their children's lives. Their parents' decision to leave Bobby's drawings and pictures in place leaves them exposed in Johnny's and Melanie's worlds, too. Ed and Elise may give the children freedom to enter Bobby's room or sift items in the garage, or they may forbid it. Ed and Elise may include them in the sorting process, offer them specific items as keepsakes, or give them opportunity to select whatever they want, or they may dispose of things without thinking of Johnny or Melanie. Similarly, Ed and Elise may decide not to return to their usual summer vacation spot without consulting the children.

Bobby's presence has touched the worlds of his grandparents to a lesser degree. Still, objects and places challenge them, and their access to some of those objects and places is even more restricted than either Johnny's or Melanie's. They now experience their own photographs and mementos in a new light. They hesitate to visit Ed's and Elise's home, dread approaching the bedroom where the accident took place, and understand Elise's reluctance to come to their home with Ed. They hesitate to return to the places where they took Bobby when his parents left him with them or where they visited as an extended family.

The neighborhood home of his best friend, a place where he spent so many hours in delightful play, holds a prominent place in David's physical environment. At times, in youthful disbelief that death is permanent, he longs to return there to play with Bobby. At other times, given what he witnessed there, he experiences nightmares or flashbacks and runs in tears to his mother. Mostly, he avoids looking at his dead friend's house. To his parents' surprise, he clings to them desperately when they take him for familiar activities outside the home. Guns and other action toys at home distress him, and now all-too-real action scenes on television terrify him. Toys that he and Bobby had shared and places where he and Bobby played make him very uncomfortable. He feels safest close to his mother, and his nightmares lead to his sleeping in the same room, sometimes in bed with his parents. His not having the words to explain why he is upset compounds his distress.

Different objects and places challenge each of us differently when we grieve. Sometimes the same objects and places challenge individuals differently. The experiences of those who knew Bobby suggest that the challenges we face vary with such things as how much we and the deceased inhabited the same space, the nature and depth of our relationship with the deceased, the circumstances of the death, and the extent to which we control interaction with the objects and places.

The range of objects and places that challenge us is perhaps most affected by the nature of our relationship to the deceased. Objects and places like those in Ed's and Elise's experiences challenge parents when they lose young children; different objects and places that matter to children as they mature challenge parents of older (including adult) children who die. Grandparents face very similar, though not identical, challenges with nearly the same objects and places.

If Ed or Elise died, the range of objects and places to be coped with and the challenges they would present to a surviving spouse would be substantially different. Anyone who loses a spouse must cope with such objects as clothing worn on special occasions, colognes and perfumes, the shared bed, items saved for and purchased, a house, the car driven to work or to a vacation retreat, gifts from the spouse, and places such as the rooms where the deceased and the surviving spouse were intimate, the town where they first met, the schools and churches they attended, and the sites of the best and worst times of their lives.

The range of objects and places to be faced and the challenges they present are also different for surviving children. Surviving children need to cope with such objects as the home where they were sheltered, the parent's favorite chair, tools in the garage or kitchen, or desk in the den or bedroom, and shared sports equipment or games. They must also face places such as those where the deceased parent sat at the dinner table, taught them to ride a bicycle, shared stories of the child's early years, offered important advice or guidance, or read them to sleep.

We Relearn Our Relationships with Fellow Survivors

Few personal relationships in his survivors' lives remain untouched by Bobby's death. Ed and Elise must cope with their profoundly strained relationship and interact with Johnny and Melanie in their grief. Ed's wife is now a bereaved parent, as is Elise's husband. What does caring require, and of what caring is each capable? Patterns of normal interaction between them seem strange, many seem inappropriate. For now they choose to sleep separately, and they avoid all but the minimal conversation necessary to carry them through the day. They anticipate that there are many conversations to be had in the future, but they choose not to begin them now for fear of compounding the tensions between them. Johnny and Melanie have now lost a brother at important stages in their personal development. How must Ed's and Elise's continued caring for them take that fact into account? How are they to find the energy and motivation to continue parenting in the midst of their own grief? Elise hopes that others in the support group will have ideas about specific things she can do or say that might help her children.

Bobby's death also affects Ed's and Elise's relationships with their own parents, in-laws, and brothers and sisters. Each interaction with another person is a task in itself. Each family member has new needs and makes new demands that combine with old but still operative expectations, and each responds to Ed's and Elise's needs and demands quite idiosyncratically. Each survivor relearns part of an experiential world of his or her own. Ed's relationships with his mother- and father-in-law, who had warned against purchase of the gun that killed their grandson, present challenges. Elise's parents may respond to Ed either as a murderer not entitled to his own grief or as a grief-stricken parent not to be condemned for his ill-advised decision. And, of course, his interactions with them will not take place entirely independently of his interactions with Elise, their daughter. For now, Ed and Elise choose to steer clear of meetings with them, fearing the worst.

Friends or acquaintances may grieve less intensely (or not at all), but many struggle with what to do and say in response to Ed's and Elise's grieving. Complication and stress fill the relationship with David's parents. Again, they choose for now to avoid contact. Some friends with children shy away from them as their loss reminds them of their vulnerability. Elise joins the support group in part to find the help and comfort she hopes for but does not receive from friends. The relief and comfort she finds there leads her to think Ed could also benefit from participating, but she hasn't yet decided how best to persuade him to try it. The death strains Ed's relationships on the job. Some coworkers avoid discussing Bobby's death, while others confront it. The utter inability of any of them to understand what Ed is going through or to comfort him makes him irritable and tries the others' patience. Elise becomes well aware that Bobby's absence transforms even relationships with service personnel, such as grocers, pharmacists, and garage mechanics. Questions such as "Have you any children?" complicate making new acquaintances. Ed and Elise are surprised at the difficulty they experience interacting with others with children Bobby's age or with anyone who reminds them of Bobby.

In their turns, Johnny and Melanie must relearn their social worlds as bereaved siblings; they must reinvent their relationships with their parents and their grandparents, each other, friends and acquaintances, and others they haven't even met. Their roles and expectations in these relationships differ markedly from those of their parents, hold distinct places in their lives, and have different meanings for them. They are anxious about whether their grieving parents will continue to provide for them. They need their parents' protection and love, yet they protect their parents from knowing how intensely they grieve. The earlier discussion of the possibility that their parents will make decisions about things and places without consulting them has obvious additional implications for their ongoing relationships with their parents. Melanie, only eleven, may be far more reluctant to protest some parental decisions that either neglect her or make it harder for her to relearn her world on her own terms. Though she wept openly when told of Bobby's death, she now hides her tears from her parents, preferring instead to cry herself to sleep at night. Her parents' obvious hurt and their emotional distance distress her nearly as much as Bobby's death itself. As a sixteen-year-old who seeks his own independent identity, Johnny does not reach out to his parents (or to anyone else for that matter) for help. He is very angry at his father for having bought the gun, but he tries not to show it. Johnny and Melanie recognize each other's hurt, but neither talks to the other about what is most distressing. They had heard their grandparents' warnings about the gun, dread a confrontation with their father and a possible division between their parents, and fear that new restrictions will be imposed by their increasingly protective parents and grandparents. None of their friends has lost someone so close, and they feel awkward and conspicuous as they return to school. Their friends often disappoint as they do not know what to do or say or simply avoid them altogether.

David's social world greatly constricts as he stays close to his parents and relies heavily on them for support, although doing so does not relieve the anxiety and terror he cannot voice. They protect him but do not know how to help him. He overhears their conversations about Bobby's parents, and the intensity of their anger worries him. He refuses to attend school, and he thereby loses contact with his other friends. Seeing how distressed he is, David's parents bring him for professional counseling, where he must learn how to interact with a virtual stranger. The counselor comforts him and lets his mother stay in the room while they play, draw, and sometimes talk.

Different relationships challenge us differently when we grieve. The experiences of those who knew Bobby suggest that the challenges vary with such factors as the qualities that characterized our relationships prior to the death, such as closeness, trust, openness, supportiveness, dependence, or ambivalence; the beliefs and emotions aroused in us by the circumstances of the death, such as anger and guilt about possible responsibility for the death; our own developmental maturity and that of those in the relationships with us; and the history and nature of our relationships to the deceased prior to the death.

The story of Bobby's death illustrates how the way survivors go about relearning the social world varies with their relationship to the deceased and the place of that relationship within their social worlds. The story traces the experiences of the newly bereaved parents, grandparents, siblings, and friends of a small child. Had the child been older, or an adult, relearning their social world would have been different since relationships with older children are different; children play different roles in families, friendships, and larger communities as they mature; and they make and receive different contributions in interactions with them.

Relearning the social world is different still when it is a spouse or companion, parent, sibling, or friend who dies. The challenges vary with the distinct characters of survivors' relationships with those who have died; the roles played by the deceased in those relationships; the nature of the give-and-take in those relationships; and the places those relationships held in the survivors' broader social networks.[6]

We Relearn Our Selves

Relearning our selves and the patterns of caring that define us as individuals is tantamount to reintegrating our selves. None of Bobby's closest survivors remain unchanged within themselves following his death. His death challenges some of them to relearn their self-identities and reinterpret their autobiographies and challenges others to understand better their limits and vulnerabilities (indeed, their mortality). Some are pressed to draw on and develop their coping capacities; others must recover their self-esteem and self-confidence, at least to the extent that these derived from give-and-take with Bobby. All must adapt their daily routines. Most must adjust the patterns of caring that define them as individuals and include caring about Bobby and what he cares about; many must reexamine their goals, hopes, and aspirations; some are moved to examine the viability of their most cherished beliefs and convictions.

Bereavement challenges us as adults to modify through grieving our typically more fully developed views of, and ways of being, ourselves. By contrast, children typically bring only tentative or prefigured views of, and are still learning how to be, themselves when bereavement short-circuits their development, compounds the challenges of learning how to be themselves, and shakes their immature senses of self-confidence and self-esteem. David, age six, is still learning whether the world outside his home is safe and trustworthy when he witnesses the shooting of his very first friend. Melanie, eleven, is learning that little girls become women and perhaps one day give birth to children like Bobby, when she both loses her little brother and witnesses the shattering effects of bereavement on her mother. Johnny, at sixteen, feels typical teen tensions with his father as he struggles to find his own identity; their relationship is complicated when Bobby shoots himself with a gun purchased by his father.

I discuss the impact of grief on personal integrity and wholeness in Chapter 5. Here I will only indicate that relearning the self at the subjective center of the world of our experience is a core part of grieving and emphasize that the challenges to relearn the self vary considerably. One source of variation is the type of relationship with the deceased. Whether we are parents, grandparents, spouses, children, grandchildren, siblings, or friends, for examples, we must, each in our own way, derive some sense of personal identity from, and flourish differently in, our relationships with those who have died.

"I am Bobby's mother," "I am Bobby's grandmother," "I am Ed's wife," "I am Elise's daughter," "I am Bobby's brother," and "I am Bobby's best friend" all declare something important but quite different about these persons' senses of who they are. Each relationship involves a different pattern of give-and-take, caring, and sharing; has different meanings; holds a different place in the life history of the survivor; and affects survivor self-confidence and self-esteem differently.

We Relearn Our Places in Space and Time

Though doctors attend to Bobby in the very next room, Ed and Elise find themselves far too remote from Bobby as they await the doctor's word. The trip home to Johnny and Melanie covers but a few blocks, yet they experience it as one of the longest journeys of their lives. When told of Bobby's death, Johnny retreats from the uncomfortable closeness he feels with his father at that moment to the open space outdoors. In contrast, both Melanie and David seek closeness as they retreat to their mother's arms. While within a few feet of those who care most about him, Ed experiences profound distance from Elise and virtual isolation in his grief at the funeral. Elise's friends' reluctance to share memories of Bobby in order not to hurt her makes them more remote. David's world constricts as he recoils from risking adventure and seeks its safest corners. The places of ordinary activity, including the workplace, are where they always have been, yet Ed, Elise, Johnny, and Melanie experience them and the everyday routine they represent as remote from their current concerns. As they yearn and search for Bobby, seeking him out in familiar places, hoping to catch glimpses of someone who looks like him, his survivors probe spaces where caring and concern now fail to find their object. Especially poignant are their attempts to find places where they sense that Bobby is close, for example, at the cemetery and, for Elise, in his bedroom and at church.

Ed and Elise experience the wait in the hospital after the accident as interminable, even though the clock registers but forty minutes of waiting time. Similarly, Ed's experiences of Elise's awkward silences have little to do with how long they last by the clock. Early in their grieving, Ed and Elise find the memory of the immediate past overwhelming as they experience devastating pain and confusion and but dimly see even the most immediate future. Ed and Elise welcome the memories aroused by the drawings and photos. Ed for now avoids the memories stored in Bobby's bedroom and beneath the blanket in the garage. Elise welcomes them in the bedroom despite the pain they arouse. Ed projects few hopes far into the future, so absorbed is he in guilt over the past. Elise sees this in him, senses his need for forgiveness, but is at a loss as to how to approach him, given what seems to her a residue of unexpressed anger. She takes hopeful steps as she attends church faithfully and joins the support group, and these activities prompt her to greater hope about Ed. Still, she is at a loss as to what to do or say that might help him to find forgiveness.

Though it has not yet occurred to any of them, Bobby's birthday and holidays, such as Halloween, Thanksgiving, Christmas, and the Fourth of July, as well as the anniversary of his death, will challenge his survivors each year. Relearning any one such occasion comprises a cluster of tasks, including deciding whether to acknowledge or celebrate at all, to retain past patterns of behavior or to modify them, choosing what to express and how to express it, and deciding whether or how to acknowledge Bobby's absence. Other significant occasions will present distinctive challenges of their own, for example, Ed's and Elise's anniversary, birthdays, Johnny's or Melanie's graduation days and the births of their own children, and David's first birthday party, which he expected Bobby to attend. Each survivor struggles with cherished memories of events peculiar to his or her private interactions with Bobby. Bobby is not alive to experience special events that are part of normal personal development (some precisely dateable and some not). However, his survivors may grieve when those events would have taken place—when he would have attended a school dance, graduated from school, taken his first job, or married.

Analysis of the spatial and temporal dimensions of the world as we experience it yields additional insights. As we relearn our worlds, we reorient ourselves within lived space and lived time. We do not experience space as a three-dimensional geometrical coordinate system or as a container that is objectively given and filled with physical objects and other persons. Similarly, we do not experience time as the regular, measured time of the clock, a string of disconnected instants. Space and time are dimensions within which we orient ourselves and assign places to objects and other persons with reference to our cares, concerns, projects, and everyday undertakings. Within the lived space of human care we experience things, places, and persons as near or remote, not more or less distant by some objective measure. Within the lived time of human care and concern we experience past, present, and future as inseparable and interpenetrating phases of personal life history. Thus, reorienting ourselves within lived space and time is an aspect of relearning both physical and social surroundings and our places within them.

As we relearn our physical and social surroundings, our tasks include recovering or establishing acceptable or comfortable spatial orientation and distance with particular objects, places and persons. The story of Bobby's survivors is replete with instances of their choosing what and whom to approach or avoid as they live in their homes and neighborhoods and venture out into the wider community.

Our tasks also include recovering or establishing acceptable or comfortable temporal orientation and distance as we come to terms with memories, hopes, and aspirations associated with particular objects, places, and persons. We reorient ourselves in time as we discern the meanings of our past life with those who have died and the events surrounding the death, test new patterns of caring involvement in present living, and seek new hope for the future. We relearn our unfolding life histories in the light of our losses. In so doing, we reinterpret and appropriate new understandings of, and come to live differently in relation to, our own past, present, and future. We also relearn especially significant events and occasions as we reinterpret their significance and learn how to live through them without the deceased.

We Relearn Our Spiritual Places in the World

Ed and Elise both feel that they do not fit in the world with Bobby gone. Both feel helpless in the face of Bobby's death. Clearly, the gun did not provide the safety and security Ed was seeking when he purchased it. Elise feels herself a victim in a threatening world. Both find it hard to go on with daily life, and neither finds meaning in any normal activity. Ed sees no end to the pain in his future, and Elise finds it hard to recover hope and aspiration for her family. Ed feels abandoned by a God he does not understand. Doing what he thought was his duty to protect his family has killed his little son. Elise cannot help but feel cheated in a world out of control. She continues attending church to find the consolation and comfort she feels she needs and to try to understand better how children's suffering is compatible with God's goodness. Despite feeling abandoned, Ed senses that he is neither ready for nor worthy of the comfort or consolation that Elise finds in church. Both go to Bobby's grave regularly in part as another way of finding a spiritually comfortable place in the world. It is doubtful that they will find comfort, consolation, or peace unless they adjust their beliefs about whether God has abandoned or punished them and about whether the world is a place where events like Bobby's death happen randomly and arbitrarily. Both struggle as they ask what kind of world it is where young children like Bobby suffer and die, as they wonder what meanings his six-year life might have, and as through their grief they recover their abilities to appreciate how Bobby touched them both in that brief life.

As we grieve, we struggle to find our place in the world in a spiritual sense.[7] Not only do we orient ourselves and our particular experiences and activities in lived space and time; we also orient the whole of our lives within the ultimate context of what we experience as the greater scheme of things. As we orient ourselves in this way, we learn, and then take for granted, how to live with at least minimal confidence that the world is a place where we and others belong and are appropriately at home. Similarly, we find confidence that the world is safe and orderly. We find ways to believe that there is a point to going on day to day, caring, pursuing purposes, hoping and aspiring, because living a human life is ultimately meaningful and worthwhile. Finally, we find confidence that there is a reason for our having the opportunity to experience, and act in, the world, however mysterious or elusive that reason may be.

Loss through death often shakes our spiritual confidence. As we grieve, we relearn our place in the world as we struggle to overcome feelings of being dislodged, uprooted, estranged, or alienated from or within the world and once again to feel we belong or are "at home" there. We seek to recover a sense of safety and security, to stop feeling fearful, anxious, vulnerable, buffeted, victimized, helpless, or powerless in a threatening world where terrible things happen to us. We struggle to overcome frustration and despair and to believe that our lives can yet be meaningful and worthwhile in a world that is hospitable to our goals, purposes, hopes, and aspirations. Finally, we struggle to experience the world once again as reasonable and orderly, rather than as chaotic, unpredictable, out of control, arbitrary, or even unfair.

Some of us recover a sense of spiritual place in passing as we relearn our worlds and establish new life patterns within them through addressing the varieties of tasks I have outlined. As we recover what remains viable in, and add new elements to, our life patterns, we settle into, and feel once again at home in, transformed places in the world. In straightforwardly coping and finding life again meaningful and purposeful, we find reassurance and make peace with the world.

For some of us, this spiritual accommodation to a world transformed by loss requires that we adjust our beliefs about the nature of the world, the (possibly divine) forces that operate within it, and the places and meanings of life, death, and suffering. At issue is the potential for meaningful life (in general or in our own cases) in a human condition pervaded by limitation, change, vulnerability, mystery, and uncertainty. Through self-conscious examination of belief, prayer, meditation, or other means, we may be able to deepen previously taken-for-granted religious faiths or secular convictions and adopt postures in the world that are more firmly rooted in the deepened convictions or faiths; others of us change faith or conviction and adopt new postures in the light of the change. Some of us achieve faiths or convictions that provide plausible answers to the questions we ponder; others among us come to faiths or convictions that enable them better to tolerate living without such answers. Where the convictions or faiths include beliefs about the divine, it is plausible to suggest that as we relearn our spiritual place in the world, we also relearn our relationships with God.

As we struggle to place our own lives in their ultimate context, we often find faiths or convictions that enable us to place the lives of the deceased in an acceptable context. The views and postures we adopt may bring comfort, consolation, and peace about the ultimate meanings and value of the life now ended. For some of us, these views and postures include beliefs about literal or symbolic immortality, in which the deceased live on in some other form or place or death does not cancel the meanings and values of their lives. Such beliefs comfort, console, or bring peace to us as survivors. And they enable those of us who hold them to sustain relationships with the deceased in their absence.[8]

The Power of the Relearning Idea

The Idea Provides General Understanding

When we, like Ed and Elise, are bereaved, our losses disrupt our ways of experiencing and living in the world that we have learned previously and come to take for granted. We lose our bearings and feel at a loss as to how to go on. We have lost not only the presence of the one who has died but much of what we took for granted. Our losses shake our confidence in potentially everything else that we also took for granted. As we cope with losses through death, we relearn what remains trustworthy in what we took for granted; where our old ways are no longer viable, we learn new life patterns. As we relearn our ways in the worlds of our experience, we find new ways of going on in the absence of those who have died, including new ways of living and being ourselves.

Viewing grieving as relearning gives specific content to the active, task-based idea of grieving and defines the range of activities involved. As we grieve, we actively engage in relearning that is not simply a cognitive affair. Instead, we engage as whole persons as we learn how to be and act in the world that is transformed by our losses. We reshape all facets of our lives.

The concept that we must relearn the world as we grieve captures both the variety and the potentially all-encompassing scale of the tasks we face. When we grieve, we must relearn virtually every object, place, event, relationships with others, and aspects of ourselves that the lives of those who have died have touched. Our grieving takes as long as it does because there is so much we must relearn. Where, when, and how the deaths will take on fresh significance is unpredictable, but it is reasonable to expect episodes of grieving through the rest of our lives. None of us does, or indeed can, encounter, or come to terms with the world all at once; what we do encounter can present new challenges later in our lives.

Seeing grieving as relearning the world provides not only a descriptively accurate but a generally applicable and broadly accessible understanding of grieving that can ground our understanding of others and of ourselves. As survivors, each of us must relearn the world in our own ways in particular circumstances. Learning is an idea familiar to nearly all of us who seek to understand grieving, not an esoteric concept accessible only to a few specially trained professionals.

Seeing that each of us is a subject at the center of a world of experience with individually unique contours underscores how each of our selves and lives is unfathomably rich, complex, and essentially never finished. Because of this, our relearning the world— our grieving—is a never-ending process that entails repeated and inevitable struggles with finiteness, continuous change, pervasive uncertainty, and vulnerability. In this open-ended coping we can glimpse the mystery of living as a self that ultimately limits others' understanding of us and our own self-understanding.

The Idea Promotes Respect for Individuality

The view of grieving as relearning fosters respect for individuality, because it emphasizes how each of us is a subjective center of a unique unfolding experience of the world. No two of us as survivors engages with the same objects, places, events, or other persons. Nor do any two of us share the same history of experiences, though to be sure our life histories do significantly intersect and overlap. No two of us have lived or been in the same relationship with those who have died. No two of us bring the same perspectives to our experiences of the world (the notion of perspective here encompasses all the elements of the taken-for-granted in our experience that I discussed earlier). No two of us bring the same predispositions in coping. Still, the general understanding of the dimensions of relearning the world that I have outlined provides entree into dialogue with any one of us when we are bereaved. Respect for any one of us as a survivor requires learning of our unique life histories and ways of experiencing, acting in, connecting with, and caring about the world around us. It requires learning what challenges us as individuals as we cope with, or relearn, virtually everything in the worlds of our experience. We grieve as individuals by meeting and addressing such specific and idiosyncratic challenges and tasks. Without knowledge of such details of our experiences, other people's understanding our individual grieving remains utterly superficial and incomplete, and respect for us as individuals is impossible.

The Idea Addresses Our Helplessness

As it places the responsibility for grief work in our own hands and undermines the plausibility of having others doing it for us, the concept of grieving as relearning the world addresses our helplessness. As we grieve, we must appropriate new ways of being ourselves in the worlds of our experience as they are transformed by our losses. No one can express our emotions, modify our self-identities, or rebuild our self-confidence and self-esteem for us. No one can change our dispositions, motivations, habits, and behaviors in our stead. No one can provide the energy or endure the physical stress that our coping requires or reestablish biological bonds with others for us. No one can take our places in interactions with others or change our relationships as our losses demand. No one can modify our perspectives, discern meanings, or adapt faiths for any of us. Just as no one can do our learning for us, neither can others lift the burden of grieving from our shoulders. We can relearn our worlds only in the first person.

The Idea Provides Guidance for Caregivers

The concept of grieving as relearning the world provides guidance for us when we wish to comfort and support those among us who are grieving. To begin, the fact that no one can learn for another defines a clear limit to our caregiving. Stated more positively, as caregivers we support and facilitate others as they themselves relearn the worlds of their experience. As caregivers we can help them recognize and address the tasks of relearning elements of their physical and social worlds as well as aspects of themselves. We can reassure the bereaved that they need not meet all challenges or address all tasks at once. We can help them focus their attention and prioritize tasks. We can encourage them to pace themselves. We can support them as they prepare for or plan to address specific tasks. We can protect their privacy or provide company as they address the tasks. And we can support them after they undertake particularly challenging tasks as we listen, help them to assess their success, and comfort, reassure, and encourage them.

As mourners address specific tasks in relearning their physical surroundings, their social worlds, and aspects of themselves, we as caregivers can support and encourage them in any or all of the facets of their coping, depending on where help and support is requested or most needed.

Psychologically and emotionally, we can help persons cope with the emotions the tasks arouse as we listen actively, normalize the feelings, empathize and comfort, encourage satisfying or meaningful expression of emotion, and tolerate those expressions. As caregivers we can help them cope with changing personal identities by providing support as they puzzle over who they are now that their loved one has died, return to familiar roles and ways of doing things, or try new roles and unfamiliar ways of doing things. We can help survivors recover or sustain self-confidence by providing reassurance as they either test still viable life patterns or build new ones. And we can support self-esteem by showing that we welcome their presence in the family or community and still value their contributions.

Behaviorally, we can support persons in making the two kinds of accommodations to loss that relearning requires. Where relearning the world involves discovering that some patterns of living remain viable after a death, we as caregivers can encourage and support testing of, and recovery of confidence in, familiar dispositions, motivations, habits, and behaviors. We can also help survivors recognize when old dispositions, motivations, habits, or behaviors lead to frustration and obstruct progress in grieving. Where relearning involves adopting new patterns of living, our helping involves supporting others as they identify options and alternatives, gather information about and evaluate the options and alternatives, choose from among them, enact those choices, and evaluate the viability of the choices once enacted.

Physically and biologically, we can help persons recognize and meet their physical needs for food, rest, and shelter as they grieve. When grief work exhausts them or overwhelms them physically, we can support the cautious use of sedatives and comparable measures, with the purpose always being to maintain health and to sustain the energy needed to cope effectively. We can also reinforce personal bonds with the bereaved by our simple presence, touch, comfort, and reassurance of their worth. And we can encourage others to offer the same rather than to compound feelings of abandonment. We can also help survivors to see that bonds with the deceased need not be thought of as completely severed.[9]

Socially, we can support persons as they reconfigure patterns of interacting with others, including family, friends, acquaintances, persons at work, or others in the wider community. As caregivers we can help the bereaved maintain relationships with others. We can support them as they anticipate and rehearse conversations and other interactions. We can offer to be with them in especially challenging social circumstances. If they wish, we can help them to avoid, deflect, or otherwise effectively deal with insensitive, disrespectful, or destructive actions of others. We can offer to intercede with others and support them if they need to break off relationships with others temporarily or permanently. We can support them as they develop new relationships. And, we can encourage them as they seek help from individuals, support groups, or professionals.

Intellectually and spiritually, we can support the bereaved as they modify understandings and perspectives, seek new meanings, or adapt beliefs and faiths. As caregivers we can help them to gather, sort, and interpret information about events surrounding the death itself. We can help them to learn more in general about the predictable impacts of bereavement and the nature and variety of tasks in grieving. If they wish better to understand themselves, we can support them as they become more self-aware and self-reflective about what has befallen them, the challenges they face and the tasks they must address in relearning their worlds, their own strengths and limitations in coping, and their own desires and hopes about what coping will bring about in their lives. We can support survivors as they modify the direction of their life histories. We can help them to recover old, and discover new, goals and purposes in day-to-day life and hopes and aspirations for the future. We can support them as they explore their understandings of and beliefs about the meanings of death, life, or suffering in general, in their individual lives, or in the lives of the deceased. And we can support them as they seek security, peace, consolation, and a return to feeling at home in the world despite human limitation and vulnerability and the mystery that pervades the human condition.

For some, personal development is incomplete or compromised. Here our caregiving involves providing additional support wherever there are developmental deficits. The challenges of grieving are especially compounded for children who experience bereavement while still effectively in the midst of "learning the world" for the first time. They are disadvantaged in emotional and psychological development as their emotional experience is limited. Their self-identities are at best in formative stages, and their self-confidence and self-esteem are fragile. They lack experience in giving direction to their own lives, either straightforwardly or self-consciously. They depend on others to meet their physical needs and are often in the midst of testing the trustworthiness of bonds with others when death occurs. They depend socially on others, who often decide paternalistically "what is best" for them, treat them as islands of innocence on the misconception that they do not grieve, and exclude them from social events such as funerals. They lack the cognitive resources to understand events surrounding the death, bereavement and grieving, and the changes in their surrounding worlds and within themselves. And they lack the spiritual resources to discern the meanings of death, life, and suffering. Nevertheless, for children, as for others, the world as they experience it is different in the aftermath of loss. As we care for them as they grieve, we must adjust our support for them in meeting the challenges by taking such developmental differences into account.

Notes

1. Alfred Lord Tennyson, "In Memoriam A.H.H.," reprinted in *The Oxford Book of Death*, ed. D. J. Enright (New York: Oxford University Press, 1983), p. 105.

2. Colin Murray Parkes suggests that coming to terms with loss, that is, grieving, is best understood as a process of relearning the world. In the remainder of this chapter and in the chapters to follow, I take that suggestion seriously.

3. In what follows, I draw heavily upon Martin Heidegger's account of human experience in its emphasis upon the distinctive character of pre-theoretical, existential involvement in the world as care, his existential concept of the worldhood of the world, and his notions of lived space and lived time. I shall not, however, be concerned to anchor the discussion in extensive textual reference and the like. See Heidegger, *Being and Time*, trans. John Macquarrie and James M. Robinson (New York: Harper and Row, 1962).

4. Colin Murray Parkes in "Psycho-Social Transitions: A Field for Study," *Social Science and Medicine* 5 (1971): 101–115, self-consciously departs from what he calls "the traditional disease-oriented field of psychiatry" and calls for study of psychosocial transitions, including grieving, wherein persons are challenged to make major changes in their "assumptive worlds" and in their surrounding life environment. He expands upon this idea in "Bereavement as a Psycho-Social Transition," *Journal of Social Issues* 44 (1988): 53–65. The work in this chapter is offered in the spirit of that work.

5. See Chapter 2 for fuller treatment of the emotion grief.

6. As I argue that the self is essentially social, in Chapter 5 I implicitly expand upon the theme of relearning social surroundings.

7. This section may be perceived as being as much about relearning the self as it is about relearning the surrounding world. And so it is. I have chosen to treat the subject here, rather than in Chapter 5, with an emphasis upon the experiences of the place of the self in the surrounding world. The theme is one of the fundamental orientation of the self to the world as the world is experienced by the self.

8. This theme of grieving as involving coming to a new relationship with the deceased in their absence is treated in a sustained way in Chapter 6.

9. Again, see Chapter 6.

5

Relearning Our Selves:
Grief and Personal Integrity

Man is but a network of relationships,
and these alone matter to him.
Antoine de Saint-Exupéry

When spider webs unite,
they scare away the lions.
Hindu proverb

I do not believe that sheer suffering teaches. If
suffering alone taught, all the world would be wise
since everyone suffers. To suffering must be added
mourning, understanding, patience, love, openness
and the willingness to remain vulnerable.
Anne Morrow Lindbergh

David's Story

When Bobby died of his gunshot wound (see Chapter 3), his best
friend David, in the room with him when the gun went off, felt
profoundly hurt, frightened, and disoriented, though he lacked
words to express himself. His parents, Bruce and Barbara, recognized his fright in his nightmares and his clinging to them but failed
to appreciate the extent and the nature of his hurt and disorientation. Barbara suspected that the event would be pivotal in David's
development, but she was not sure of its long-term effects.

When Bobby died David was an unprecocious, friendly six-year-
old boy. Bruce and Barbara loved him and in most ways were still the

This chapter greatly expands and develops an earlier essay, "Grief and Personal
Integrity," in *Priorities in Death Education and Counseling* (Hartford: Forum for
Death Education and Counseling, 1982).

center of his life. He had attended half-day kindergarten the year before, was an eager first-grader, and was starting to make friends outside his neighborhood. He was becoming comfortable moving beyond the narrow physical and social confines of his early life, learning to do things in school and at play, and feeling good about himself and the happy experiences and adventures that filled his days. He wished that his mother would trust him without checking on him so often, looked forward to learning to ride his new Christmas bicycle, and was excited about how he secretly explored the neighborhood and a little beyond with Bobby. His best friends lived in the neighborhood, and his parents did not let him venture far from the block without supervision. Bobby had moved next door when both were three years old, and he played more with Bobby than with all his other friends combined. They vowed to live near each other always, dreamed of being baseball players, and doubted that either would ever have any interest in girls.

Bobby's death traumatizes David. Not only does he hear the shot; he sees the bullet enter Bobby's body and the bleeding and hears Bobby cry and moan. In the midst of the chaos, others virtually ignore his trauma. Bobby's mother, Elise, says nothing to him and little to Barbara as she rushes him home while Ed, Bobby's father, brings Bobby to the car to go to the hospital. David blurts out a quick explanation to his mother that Bobby shot himself and then melts into tears in her arms. Though he wants to go to Bobby's funeral, Bruce and Barbara think he hurts too much already and refuse to take him. They also fear what they might say to Ed and Elise, given how angry they are with them over the incident. David never sees Bobby after the shooting. In the next few weeks, David has many nightmares, refuses to return to school, loses contact with other friends, clings to Bruce and Barbara, worries about their intense anger at Bobby's parents, and eventually, at Barbara's insistence, is brought to a professional counselor by his parents, who sense that he needs help they do not know how to offer.

David's counselor works with the image of the death scene that haunts him and disrupts his sleep. He uses art therapy to help David identify what frightens him so in the image, to undermine its power and hold on him, and to help him to carry the image alongside other nonthreatening images of Bobby. Within three months the nightmares disappear, and David feels safe sleeping in his own room again. His counselor helps David decide to say good-bye to Bobby as he visits his grave, leaves a toy there, and brings some drawings to Bobby's parents. He also helps David face Bobby's house next door;

stop expecting to see, or play with, Bobby; return to school; and begin, hesitantly, to find other things to do with his time and energy, such as exploring his neighborhood and again playing with friends.

David senses that his friends find him strange. He far prefers playing at home. He does not want to talk about what he has seen and heard and says so, but they don't seem to understand. He refuses to join in games with guns, even water pistols. He avoids violence in television programs, even cartoons, and video games. And he does not join in when other boys talk and laugh about things that are "gross." He senses that some boys don't play with him any more because they don't know what to do when with him. He senses that he isn't fun to be with. None of the boys is quite like Bobby, and at times his heart is not in playing with them. Only a few come for his first birthday party ever.

David is filled with questions. He wonders about so many things. "Why was Bobby shot and not me? Could Mommy or Daddy die? Could I die? What's so scary about a funeral? What's it like when you're dead? Does it hurt? When do you wake up? What do grown-ups mean when I hear them say Bobby is in heaven with Jesus? Why does God take only the best little children to be with him like Mommy says? And, if He does, why have I been left behind? Why did I have to lose my best friend when no one else did?" Because his parents refuse to let him attend Bobby's funeral or explain what it is about, and because they talk about such things only when they think he cannot hear, he senses that no one wants to answer his questions, so he keeps them to himself.

In a separate session held at the counselor's request, Bruce and Barbara learn of the counselor's efforts and about what he expects the long-term effects of Bobby's death on David's development will be. The counselor says that he has tried to help David overcome a fixation with his nightmare image, feel he has some control over his own experiences, and return to a normal life pattern for a boy who has just turned seven. He says David may find it hard to trust his parents' protection, his friendships, and the safety of his world. He notes that David may always have strong feelings about guns and violence. He cautions that David is old enough to remember vividly the trauma. It will trouble him now and again as he comes to new stages of his life and determines who he is, what he cares about, and what the meanings of his life are and can be. The counselor cannot predict the exact effects of the loss on David's development, but David surely will revisit his experience. As his coping capacities develop, each revisiting is likely to result in shifts in life pattern or self-understanding. He will need patience, understanding, and support from his parents (and, later, from others).

Margaret's Story

When her three grandchildren and her daughter Mary died (see Chapter 4), Margaret was traumatized by what she saw and frustrated in her efforts to reach out for support. Her husband, Earl, urged her to put her mind on other things and seemed quite unable to provide the support she needed. In deference to her fear that he might have another heart attack, and resigned to the inadequacies of his emotional support, Margaret held her grief within and paced the floor at night after Earl went to sleep. She held to this pattern for eight months until Earl died in his sleep of a massive heart attack, compounding her losses and leaving her a widow. Months later, in a widow-to-widow support group, she said, "It was shattering. The pain cut me to the core. Following so close on the deaths of Mary and my dear grandchildren, I felt as if I was literally falling apart. I knew I could never be the same person again, and I seriously wondered if Earl's death would destroy me. I felt as if an irreplaceable part of me were gone forever. I'm still not sure just how I'm going to make it. Thank God for you good people and what's left of my lovely family."

Margaret, fifty-eight years old at the time of the deaths, had devoted her adult life to her domestic roles as wife of Earl, mother to her seven children (including Diane and Mary), and Nana to the growing number of grandchildren (including Ann, Mike, and Jimmy, all of whom had died with Mary). She had a rich store of memories of a full adult life, lived comfortably, if a bit uneasily, with Earl, and had great hopes for her future and those of the ones she loved. Earl was very successful in his own business, and Margaret enjoyed the social life it made possible, including connections with the wives of other prominent businessmen and with civic leaders in the community.

The first deaths devastated her. Then her worst fears about Earl were realized. After his earlier heart attack, she feared for him in his bereavement and as he faced his retirement at age sixty-five, only three months after the accident. Though she had no clue as to the intensity of his feelings about the deaths and the end of his career, she sensed that both events deeply troubled and unsettled him. She wondered whether he was thinking of the nearness of his own death.

Always a man of few words, he held his own counsel and never let her know just what he was experiencing. Still, she was convinced that his silence contributed to the fatal attack.

She always straightforwardly and instinctually carried herself through even the most difficult challenges, but her instincts failed her when Mary and the young ones died. She reached out to Earl, only to be rebuffed and encouraged to simply get on with living without thinking about the deaths or what she had seen when she found the bodies. She couldn't speak with Diane about her experience because of the effect it would have on her. It seemed so unfair to burden her other children. She was embarrassed to approach her social friends because none had ever been a confidant before. She resolved, but never managed, to seek professional help.

After Earl's death, some of her friends turn away from her altogether because they are either too uncomfortable with her pain or unwilling to include her in activities for couples only. Her sleepless nights still take a terrible toll, and she feels "stuck" on a treadmill heading nowhere. She realizes that her own life expectancy is limited, and she fears that she may never again live well. She senses that she has only two choices: She can allow herself to be overwhelmed by the accumulated losses, or she can somehow turn herself around, reach out for help, and find a way of living decently well again despite the losses. Earl's death and the reminder of her own mortality push her to take unprecedented steps to care for herself.

She first approaches her minister, but he senses that he is in over his head with the problems that preoccupy her. He invites her to come back later after she sees the counseling psychologist he recommends. The psychologist immediately recognizes Margaret's needs deriving from the trauma of finding the bodies and holding all her feelings inside. She prescribes sedatives that allow Margaret to sleep through the night and fight the exhaustion that threatens to overwhelm her. She helps her to defuse the power of the traumatic vision as they vividly rehearse the details of the scene. This triggers intense, cathartic expression of her feelings and enables her gradually to change the place of the vision and the horrors it invokes in her. Similar work defuses the trauma of finding Earl dead, which reawakens the trauma of finding the first bodies. Learning to live with those scenes is the first step as Margaret recovers her equilibrium.

Margaret wrestles mightily with her ambivalent relationship with Earl. He provided well and left her with a considerable fortune from his successful career. He was a fair, if stern, father and grandfather. However, he never fully appreciated how much she sub-merged her own identity in his and the extent to which she carried the greater burdens at home. As in his business, at home he was controlling and at times nearly tyrannical. His failure to support her when Mary and the children died was not the first time he had let her down; she had long felt, but never expressed, her resentment at his not "being there" for her emotionally. His refusal even to listen to her tale of discovering the bodies particularly galled her, but she swallowed her resentment rather than risk upsetting him when it would do no good, anyway. Earl enjoyed the company of his family at the frequent clan gatherings, but she always sensed that his real love was his business. She spent many lonely nights waiting for his late return from work. In some ways she now feels lost without him, but in others she feels relief that is at first hard to admit to herself or her counselor.

Without Earl, Margaret finds it difficult to return to her nearly entirely domestic life. So much of her time seems empty. She repeatedly catches herself expecting him to drive into the garage, come through the door, sit at the dinner table, make his little messes, take an interest in what she experiences, and prepare to do things with her. So many of the little things she did to make a home for the two of them no longer make sense for one. Yet she eventually derives great satisfaction from her surviving children and grandchildren as she devotes more time and energy to them.

She returns to her minister for spiritual counseling. Her faith remains strong, but the mystery of God's ways in the world deepens for her. The minister helps her as she wonders, "Do I really belong on earth, or is my place with Earl and the children in heaven? How can I be forgiven for feeling badly about Earl the way I do? Where can I find peace and solace after such terrible things happen? Why do the young ones have to die while I linger on? What is the point of my going on?" She comes to see her own remaining years as a precious gift and resolves to do something more with them before it is too late.

When she appears ready, her psychologist recommends that she join a support group for widows, and she finds great comfort, reassurance, and friendship there, a kind of friendship and openness she has never known before. She transfers the sharing she finds there to her interaction with her family with some success, especially with her daughters and her daughters-in-law, to whom she draws closer than ever before. Other widows tell of taking bold steps to reshape their lives, and they inspire Margaret.

Though she helped Earl with some money management in the

early days, she has neither formal training nor experience in work outside the home. A career seems out of the question. She thinks it too late for school and is too proud to begin "at the bottom." A corporate attorney friend presents the idea that leads her to strike out in a new direction in life. He has made the arrangements himself, and he reminds her that the futures of the children and grandchildren are well assured through trust funds. She has a fortune big enough to provide well for herself, be generous with the family, and still have a great deal left over. He suggests that she explore using the money to contribute to the community. She mulls the idea, talks it over with Bill, Diane, and her other children, and goes with Bill to speak with her friend and his associates about establishing a foundation to support projects to serve children. The foundation will start with funds from her fortune, and some of Earl's professional associates will manage its business operations. She will name it for Earl and dedicate it in loving memory of the children. She will exploit her social connections for sources of additional funding, publicize the foundation, and review proposals. Once projects are under way, she will visit the children and those who help them and, as she puts it, "extend her family even further." She finds it a worthy legacy for Earl and the children and a way to sense she is making a difference. She experiences herself as extending her efforts "to do God's work" into the broader community.

How Are We to Understand Ourselves in Loss and Grief?

Both David and Margaret change utterly in and through their experiences of loss. When we are bereaved, like Margaret, we often describe our loss experiences as shattering. Some of us, like David, may not use those words, but the description fits with our experiences of who we are. We sense that we can never be the same persons we were prior to our losses. Profound changes in our worlds seem to call for profound changes in us, changes that many of us do not well understand and that often frighten us. Frequently, we are surprised at the nature and intensity of the effects of personal loss. Self-doubt often accompanies our surprise as we wonder whether we are alone in feeling such anguish and whether we will ever be whole again.

Common discussions of bereavement and grieving tell us little about our selves and our personal integrity that can help us understand our anguish over the shattering effects of bereavement or the anguish of others whom we would support and comfort. What is it to be a self? How may we usefully think of our personal integrity?

How do we become the selves we are? How does bereavement affect us as the individuals we have become? How is it that we experience bereavement as partial disintegration of our selves? How may our grieving be understood as a struggle to put ourselves together again? Profoundly affected by the impacts of loss, we transform our selves through grieving. As we grieve, we relearn who we are at the centers of the worlds of our experience.

How We Become the Selves We Are

Imagine a delicately woven web, much like a spider's web, attached to its surroundings at points beyond counting. Innumerable threads radiate from the center of the web, and countless transverse threads bind the radiating threads. Each radiating thread represents a way in which we, like Margaret and David, attach ourselves to the world. In reality, there are usually many threads of connection between us and the persons, places, things, and projects that matter most to us, so perhaps we should imagine a wedge of the web, or an array of radiating threads, as representing the multifaceted attachments we have with any single other person. A web representing David's life pattern would feature prominent wedges of attachment to Barbara and Bruce (his parents) and to Bobby (his best friend), with far smaller wedges for school, his other friends, and some of his projects at home. A web representing Margaret's life pattern would feature far more richly developed, multistranded wedges of attachment to Earl, her home, and her children, with smaller wedges for each of her grandchildren and still other wedges for her many friends and social contacts and for the other things that matter to her in her world.

Individual radiating threads represent the full range of particular emotional, practical, physical, social, intellectual, and spiritual ties between us and elements of the world around us, especially other persons we care about. Along those lines of connection we form bonds in patterns of give-and-take with each other. Among the many positive things that we give and receive are material assistance, help in daily efforts, information, instruction, expertise, intellectual stimulation, simple attention, advice and counsel, direction, spiritual assistance, honest feedback, perspective, candor, companionship, togetherness, sharing in activities, modeling of how to be, interest, admiration, praise, encouragement, affirmation, emotional support, expressions of confidence, reinforcement, acceptance, understanding, trust, a sense of belonging, effective listening, empathy, compassion, respect, comfort, reassurance, forgiveness, dependability, loyalty, friendship, love, emotional sharing, caring, affection, warmth, physical contact, pleasure, sexual satisfaction, and satisfaction at contributing to others' well-being. Sometimes the give-and-take in our lives is mutual; sometimes it is not. Still, we are bound as one of us gives and the other accepts what is given. As we give and receive, we form unique bonds as acquaintances, associates, friends, companions, spouses, parents and children, and siblings.

Early in his life David mostly received love, affection, and all that they entail from his parents. Only gradually has he begun to give more in return. Psychologists tell us that these first bonds with parents establish our sense of stability and trust in the world. In his first friendships, especially his friendship with Bobby, David has learned for the first time the possibilities of reciprocity with peers. This early giving and receiving establish foundations and models for later relationships.

Margaret lived with Earl for more than thirty-five years, during which time she gave and received much that typically is exchanged only within long-standing, intimate relationships. Earl's giving was not particularly warm, but it was genuine. He expressed love through constancy, devotion, and faithfulness; the intensity of his efforts to provide well; his concern for her safety, security, and well-being and for those of their children; and his appreciation for her supporting him emotionally, nurturing the children, and providing a warm, loving home environment. Her giving was emotionally generous and forgiving. She expressed her love through her constancy, devotion, faithfulness, and, often, deference to his wishes, patience with his long hours of work and admiration for his drive to succeed; appreciation for all that he provided; care for his children; and gratitude for the affection he shared with her and with them.

Give-and-take along the lines of connection between people is not always positive. Some powerful and binding connections are negative. Moreover, within any single array, some connecting threads are strong and well-established, while others are weak or frayed. Because of the complexity of the patterns of give-and-take among us, no two bonds between people are exactly alike. The web metaphor captures the complexity within our particular relationships, including the existence of negativity and ambivalence.

There was little ambivalence in David's friendship with Bobby, though they did "fight" now and again. The air was free of all such negative feelings when Bobby died. Fortunately, David never said, even in play, that he wished Bobby were dead. In contrast, the marriage between Margaret and Earl was filled with ambivalence. Earl, to some extent, gave Margaret the feeling that he was disappointed that she had not found an identity outside the home, especially after the children left. She felt that he never appreciated the extent of her self-sacrifice and her submersion of her identity in his. She was quite dependent on him, disappointed that he could not provide emotional as well as financial support, and resentful of his control over her life and that of her family. Prior to his death, she swallowed much of her anger; in fact, her habit of swallowing was so well developed that she was barely aware of the anger while Earl lived.

The transverse threads of the web represent an additional complexity in our personal life patterns. No single array of attachment to one important person in our lives is isolated from any of the others, though the connections are at times quite remote. For example, a pattern in one of our relationships with one who is very close, perhaps a spouse like Earl or one of our parents, has much to do with our relationships with other intimates, including our children and friends. It is less obvious, but nevertheless true, that the pattern of such a close relationship is linked with far more remote aspects of our life patterns, such as how we dress, what motivates us at work, what we do in a supermarket, how we spend our leisure time, where we prefer to vacation, and how we respond to others who superficially resemble a spouse or parent. Indeed, such interrelatedness pervades our attachments to the world, and these patterns are a vital key to understanding our personal integrity. The web metaphor illustrates how a change in one part of a life can affect the entire fabric of that life, although we are usually oblivious to the extent of this connection pattern. In most cases, then, it is appropriate to imagine the transverse threads of the web as translucent. You have to look closely to see them.

The metaphor also allows us to imagine our personal life histories as requiring that we perpetually weave and reweave the threads of attachment to persons, places, things, and projects in our lives. As we live our lives, we establish, broaden, enrich, combine, transform, and at times discard or abandon such attachments. For David, life is just beginning; for Margaret, the history of weaving and reweaving is long and richly developed. We may weave and reweave life patterns straightforwardly and unreflectively or self-consciously and deliberately. David has yet to develop his style, while Margaret's was, at least prior to Earl's death, straightforward. We flourish and find and achieve purpose and meaning within such patterns of caring.

We become who we are through the modes of caring that dominate our lives and the variety, breadth, and depth of our personal attachments to what we care about.

We are not born with self-concepts, self-images, self-confidence, or self-esteem. These emerge from our life histories of interaction with others and from our experiences. Psychologists tell us that at the very earliest stages of our personal development we do not differentiate between our selves and others. Early on, our *self-concepts*, or the ways we think of ourselves, derive entirely from interactions with others. There is no difference between our self-concepts and our *self-images*, or the way we perceive others as aware of us. As others give to us along lines of connection, either positively or negatively, our self-images, and through them the beginnings of our self-concepts, emerge. Our self-concepts are enriched through self-awareness as we test and develop our capacities to function and flourish through interaction with the persons, places, and things around us. As we find our own abilities to give to others, act and accomplish, our *self-confidence*, or our perceptions of our own abilities, joins our self-image to create a distinct component of our self-concept. In turn, our *self-esteem*, or our estimate of our own worth, emerges as yet another aspect of our self-concept.

Our early self-esteem derives predominantly from our accepting or rejecting the evaluations of our selves that others communicate and reinforce. Some of us (but not all) later develop the capacity for more autonomous self-evaluation (based on our self-perceived success and failure in projects and social interactions), though few of us are uninfluenced by the evaluations of others. Thus, our self-concepts, self-images, self-confidence, and self-esteem emerge as we establish distinctive webs of connection with others. Some of us find additional grounding in faith or conviction about our relationship with God or with the powers of the universe, however we conceive them.

David is at the beginning of his personal development, still very much concerned with how others think of him. Hence, he needs much reassurance from his parents. Bobby's death shakes David's nascent self-confidence, and he withdraws into the safety he knew first and best at home. He wonders whether God loves him, since He took Bobby to heaven and not him. Margaret, in contrast, is a developed adult. Prior to Earl's death she thought of herself primarily as others saw her, and her self-confidence was rooted in her successes in raising her children to adulthood. She now wonders with her minister about her worthiness in God's eyes.

Each of our *selves*, with its own identity, is the consciousness embodied in the individual patterns of caring connection with the world that emerge as we weave and reweave the webs of our lives. Our *integrity as a self* is the pattern or structure of the web, both the radiating threads and the transverse threads that bind them. Our individual *self-identity*, which emerges through the lived history of our weaving and reweaving, is the evolving, more or less coherent connection among the past, present, and future of each of our lives. Our *individuality* as selves derives from our present pattern of connection, both in the unique combinations of radiating threads and in the distinctive patterns of connection between them (the transverse threads) that are woven into the fabric of our lives. Our individuality also derives, in part, from our particular histories, through which we develop distinctive habits, dispositions, character traits and capacities; bring our individual background experiences to our present living; and project our unique hopes and dreams into the future.

The web metaphor illustrates how our identities are informed by many threads of care that secure us in the world. Our personal relationships and attachments are not accidents but rather essential components of our personal integrity and identity and are decisive in making us who we are. Moreover, our self-concepts, self-images, self-confidence, and self-esteem have fundamentally social roots. As individuals we are deeply socially embedded and interdependent in our relationships with others, and our capacities to flourish and to find purpose and meaning in life are social or socially dependent. These capacities are in large measure capacities for society. We do not develop and use them, however, unless we find partners who allow us to do so. We become the selves we are in society as we express ourselves through language, learn from and with others, join in common endeavors, make friends, share intimacy, empathize, and participate in other social interactions. Within complex give-and-take patterns we become who we are and find the support and sustenance we require to remain intact as the individuals we become.

David is who he is by virtue of his connections with his parents and friends and his activities at school. His individuality is still forming when Bobby dies. Still, he connects uniquely with others and brings some limited coping capacities to his bereavement. Margaret is a much more fully developed individual. Her connections with others are far more extensive, and the interconnections among her relationships are far more complex. She is not Earl; yet in many ways his identity has submerged hers. His place in society at large and his contributions are more prominent and recognized. She sees herself as the person who contributed most to making Earl's accomplishments possible and thinks of herself as others think of her, as wife, mother, and grandmother, that is, in terms of her giving to others.

To see the essentially social and interdependent character of our lives as individuals, imagine that the web of each of our individual lives is but one web in a huge network of webs that together make up human society. As selves, we live in near-constant interaction with others. We secure our individuality and personal integrity in the tension between and among the webs in the network. No one of us owns any of the radiant threads of connection that we establish with others. We share ownership. The encouragement, help support, or love that one of us gives is the same encouragement, help, support, or love that is received by the other. Only the transverse threads that bind radiant threads together in our particular webs are contained in just one web, but they alone do not determine our individuality. Rather, our individuality is discernible and achievable only within the history of the weaving of the large fabrics of our families, communities, and societies. The boundaries between our selves are permeable, flexible, and fluid, and the narratives of our individual lives find their distinctive contours within broader social narratives.

These broader social and historical contexts strongly influence how we develop and flourish. Where each of us is located in the broader web of webs—our particular set of life circumstances—has much to do with what patterns of give-and-take we establish along lines of connection with others. Our self-concepts, self-images, self-confidence, self-esteem, personal development, character traits and coping capacities, patterns of flourishing, personal integrity, personal identity, and individuality all are influenced by our gender, age, class, and ethnic, religious, and cultural backgrounds. In these ways, too, our selves are social and interdependent.

David, as a boy, is just beginning to feel the effects of such social influences. Men and women continue to be treated differently in society, especially when it comes to sex-role socialization. The unfortunate fascination with guns and violence in contemporary America is largely a male fascination and may have contributed to the curiosity with firearms that led to Bobby's death. Expectations of how he should deal with life's adversities, express emotions, and so on will probably affect David throughout his life. Fortunately for him, his parents at this early stage of his development are not inclined to press him to "be strong" or "get over it," as they or others might later in life. What he overhears about Jesus, God, and heaven confuses him. Perhaps later a mature faith will support him.

Margaret willingly accepted a traditional woman's role as homemaker and mother. When she grew up and made the decisions that defined the person she became, she accepted limits on the range of options she seriously entertained. She believed that a woman's fulfillment was most likely to come in domestic life. She received approval for these choices not only from Earl but also from most of her peers and from members of their parents' generation. She believed that God also condoned her choices. Her cultural heritage influenced her to be self-reliant and to call on others only rarely for help, to be uncomplaining, to refrain from burdening others with the difficulties of meeting challenges in her personal life, and to "keep the faith" no matter what adversity life might bring. Fortunately for her, with these influences well entrenched, she knew little adversity and prospered until she lost Mary, the three little ones, and then Earl.

Our Selves in Loss and Grief: Elaborating the Image

Imagine that a wedge of the web represents that part of David or Margaret that cares about, and participates in a relationship with, Bobby or Earl. Imagine the death of either, then, as a blow delivered where that wedge is anchored and penetrating to the center of the web so that loose ends hang where once there was connection. The blow dislodges all the security in the world and all the structure in the self that the relationship provided. It leaves unanchored all the desires, motivations, habits, and behaviors that were parts of the relationship. Such a disorienting blow tears at the very fabric of the grieving person. It puts David and Margaret in crisis, as it would any of us who are bereaved.

When a particular relationship holds a prominent place in our lives, a death strikes a severe blow to our personal integrity by dislodging an even broader wedge of the web. David interacts with few other people, so Bobby's loss represents a substantial loss to his network of social relationships. Margaret's interactions are far more extensive. Yet, because her ties to Earl were so varied and so central to her individuality, his death is also a severe blow. Thus, the metaphor allows us to illustrate the relative severity of a particular loss. It also demonstrates how multiple losses, especially if occurring within short periods of time that allow for little mending of the web, threaten us with total disintegration. This is precisely Margaret's experience. The additional blow of Earl's death, coming so soon after her other losses, threatens complete disintegration.

It takes much weaving and reweaving to create a fully developed and well-anchored web. The history of that weaving and reweaving gives each web a unique character; a major blow undoes much of that weaving and reweaving. When someone dies, we experience ourselves as undone by the loss. The death disrupts the narrative of our shared history with the one who has died, and we are at a loss as to how to go on. The patterns of our lives as survivors are forever altered. Sometimes the experience of our own fragility in bereavement reminds us of, and moves us to reflect on, our own mortality.

Though he hasn't the words for it, it is in part this dismay over how to go on without Bobby that hurts, frightens, and disorients David. Margaret is far more aware of how her life story is intricately interwoven with Earl's, and early in her bereavement she is very much at a loss as to how to go on without him. Neither David nor Margaret can be the same as he or she was prior to the deaths, for no one can ever replace Bobby or Earl. David's private wondering about whether he, too, could die frightens him; Earl's death reminds Margaret that her own time is limited, and her reflection leads her to see the time remaining as a gift too precious to waste.

A blow reverberates throughout the structure of a web. So, too, death reverberates throughout our lives, as it does for David and Margaret. The degree and character of the reverberations varies with the severity of the blow, and with the nature and extent of the interconnectedness of personal involvements in our individual life patterns. A blow introduces new tensions throughout the web and makes new demands on all lines of connection in our lives. David's parents wonder what to do for and with him, as do Margaret's children about her. David and Margaret, in their turns, wonder how they need or want to be with their fellow survivors. Such new tensions are as unique and as varied as the distinctive patterns of caring that we establish.

Last, the tensions on transverse threads dislodge other radiating threads from their anchors at locations remote from the area where the blow has struck. For example, David no longer sees Bobby's parents on a nearly daily basis, and he fears returning to school. Margaret at first loses interest in her friends and does not discuss her grieving with her own children because she fears it will be too hurtful for them. This additional disintegration of the web represents another shattering quality of our loss experiences. We often sense that our "lives are falling apart." David senses it but lacks the words, whereas Margaret voices these feelings fully. Not only do we lose the deceased; we also experience ourselves as distanced from those around us, perhaps even from God, and as no longer firmly grounded in our everyday lives. Nothing seems quite the same, since we truly must relearn the entire world.

Just as the whole web is shaken by a localized blow, so we react to loss with our entire being. Our selves react to loss organically. Our typical initial shock and numbness are organic and pervasive. As we pull back from reality, we marshal the emotional, behavioral, physical, social, intellectual, and spiritual energies needed to cope with our new reality. This process is evident in David's retreat to the safety of home and his mother's arms and in Margaret's silence, which so frightens her children.

The web metaphor suggests that grief work and relearning of the world require more or less total reweaving of our selves. Each of our selves simply is the consciousness embodied in the patterns of our personal involvements. As David and Margaret relearn their physical and social worlds and reconstruct viable life patterns, they relearn themselves; they learn how to be who they want to be in the world as they come to terms with the residue of their relationships with the deceased. As we address the individual and innumerable tasks of coming to terms with the elements of our lives, we form new patterns of living within which we become changed persons. Depending on whether grieving goes poorly or well, our selves remain in tatters or we attain a new integrity. Ineffective grieving compromises our personal integrity and diminishes our flourishing; effective grieving brings us new resiliency and enables us to live more fully in appreciation of the place and value of connectedness in a life of integrity.

As We Cope, We Engage with and Move Beyond Suffering

It can be useful to define suffering as the experience of loss of wholeness and the distress and anguish that accompany it. When we are bereaved, we experience, to varying degrees, a loss of organic wholeness. As whole persons, we absorb the loss in all facets of our being simultaneously. The emotional impacts of our losses reflect not only our longing for emotional wholeness in reunion with those who have died but our anxiety about the possibility of again feeling whole in other relationships. We are at a loss as to what to do in our daily life where our taken-for-granted motivations, dispositions, habits, and behaviors no longer fit our reality. We experience the severing of bonds essential for our biological survival, integrity, and flourishing. We feel disconnected not only from those who have died but from our customary patterns of social interaction with our fellow survivors. Intellectually and spiritually, we no longer feel at home in the world. Like Margaret, many of us are at a loss for self-understanding as we experience major discontinuities in our life stories and do not see how coherence, hope, and meaning are still possible for us. Like David, many of us are filled with unanswered questions about what death is and why particular deaths have occurred.

When we are bereaved, we suffer loss of wholeness in three interconnected ways: Loss shatters the patterns of our present lives, disrupts the narrative flow of our autobiographies, and leaves us feeling disconnected from larger wholes of which we have thought ourselves part. As we address the tasks of grieving, we reestablish wholeness in our lives in each of these spheres. We reestablish coherence in our present living; we reestablish continuity in the ongoing stories of our lives; and we recover old meanings or find new ones in the larger wholes of which we are, or become, parts.

As we grieve, we struggle to relieve or ameliorate the distress and the anguish of suffering. In part, when we suffer we experience ourselves as passive recipients of blows to our present life patterns, disruptions in our autobiographies, and separations from larger wholes. We often experience our plight as beyond our control, our losses as irretrievable, our distress and anguish as without end, our future as hopeless, and ourselves as powerless and helpless in our suffering. Part of what so frightens David is the unprecedented helplessness he feels as he realizes that his friend, unlike cartoon characters, will not come back to life. Margaret feels vastly put upon by forces beyond her control. At first, neither sees any way that the distress and the anguish are likely to subside. Because we so often experience our suffering as inflicted from without, as unrelenting, and as unlimited in time, we tend to freeze in place in our suffering, and we are left languishing and desperate, unmotivated or unable to act.[1] David and Margaret experience this paralysis.

To reestablish wholeness in our lives, we must move beyond the paralysis of such suffering. We must believe we are not helpless and that there is some point (however obscure) in addressing the tasks of relearning our worlds; we must find the motivation to learn how to be our selves again without those who died. As we cope, we free ourselves from the immobilizing effects of lingering suffering.

Margaret's recognition of her own mortality provides powerful motivation for her active coping. David's and Margaret's counselors help them to engage actively with the traumatic visions that captivate them and contribute to their helplessness. Although our distress and anguish cannot be made to disappear, grieving is in part a transition from being fully self-absorbed and nonfunctional in distress and anguish (in an important sense, *being* them) to carrying and enduring distress and anguish (in an important sense, *having* them) as we become functional again and reestablish wholeness in our lives.[2] We must find such grief work worth the trouble. Simply moving and functioning again, often with little reason to believe it "will do any good," can start us down the road to reestablishing wholeness and overcoming suffering. While distress and anguish may remain our life's companions, they can be put into perspective within reintegrated selves that they no longer dominate. Such coping relieves our suffering.

As we grieve, we also struggle to restore what is still viable in our previously established life patterns. Much of our pre-death wholeness depended on the presence of the deceased, and this wholeness cannot be restored. But much of our life patterns may remain viable. We commonly overestimate the extent of the damage to our taken-for-granted life patterns. Despite new strains and tensions throughout our lives, we can in fact restore, or recover, much of what previously sustained us as whole selves. In this way, our coping with loss revives our selves. David's counselor and parents and Margaret's counselor and the widows in the support group move David and Margaret to engage actively with other people, things, and projects that still matter to them. David returns to school and to budding friendships. Margaret finds solace in her ongoing, albeit strained, life with her still large extended family, and she renews her faith in her visits with her minister.

As we grieve, we struggle too to transform our selves, to establish something unprecedented. At the very least, we adjust and accommodate to the absence of the deceased. Even preexisting patterns and connections that are revived or recovered are changed to this extent. However, we may establish new life patterns as we find new and unexpected ways of living. We may discern new and fresh meanings in the next chapters of our autobiographies, or we may find and build new connections with self-transcending wholes. We then become wholes we never were before. Our new wholeness often supports a new kind of flourishing and we grow or develop as persons through our loss experiences. Such coping enhances our selves. David's full development lies largely before him when Bobby dies. As he becomes the person he is capable of becoming and incorporates his loss experience into the process, he will become a whole he has never been before. As Margaret establishes the foundation and reaches out to her community, she enhances her life and, as she sees it, appreciates the gift that it is.

Unless we can move beyond paralysis in suffering, we can neither restore previously existing elements of our wholeness nor transform and establish unprecedented wholeness in our lives. Our coping with loss serves all three functions. As individuals we vary widely in our motivation and capacity to transcend our suffering as we carry the distress and anguish, reconnect, and establish new connections. We come to our loss experiences with more or less well developed coping capacities and diverse background experiences, including the legacies of other losses.[3] Moreover, our coping and reintegration of our selves is socially influenced, bounded by, and interdependent with the coping of fellow survivors (this point is discussed more fully later in this chapter).

When Bobby dies, David's abilities both to flourish and to cope with loss, like those of most children his age, are marginally developed or nearly nonexistent. He brings no legacy of previous losses to his bereavement. Margaret, in contrast, is well able to flourish in family and other relationships. She has coped with previous losses reasonably well through self-reliance and with family support. However, none of the earlier deaths was so sudden or traumatic. Her straightforward and instinctive coping proves inadequate to the challenges presented by the cluster of deaths that occurs within eight months in her fifty-ninth year. As she still grieves the losses of Mary and the children, Earl's death nearly overwhelms her.

We Struggle to Put Our Shattered Lives Back Together

Not only do David and Margaret yearn and search for Bobby and Earl; they also yearn and search for the old selves they can no longer be and for the new selves they have yet to become. David is lost in all but the narrowest regions nearest his parents. He gradually lets go of his expectations of seeing and playing with Bobby and fills the void as he begins to explore the neighborhood without him and to play with new friends. Margaret no longer fits into the domestic life in which she raised their children with, and devoted herself to, Earl, continuing to care for him when the children left to raise their own families. She feels a great emptiness in her daily life as she continues to expect Earl to be there, to do his usual things, to share experiences with her, and to join in activities. She learns to live alone in her home, do things for one rather than two, and fill her days with expanded interaction with her surviving family and with new experiences and activities with the widows' group and with the foundation.

When we are bereaved, *we experience divisions within our selves* as the webs of our lives are torn asunder. We experience ourselves as broken wholes, fragmented or shattered. The desires, motivations, dispositions, habits, behaviors, and day-to-day expectations and hopes once grounded in our relationships with those who have died still operate but now lack their taken-for-granted anchoring in the world. The pattern of our day-to-day living built around those who have died loses viability. We experience ourselves as suspended between a reality where we were at home and knew how to be ourselves and a reality transformed by loss where we have yet to find our way. The pervasive disorientation that we so often experience when we are bereaved reflects the broader pattern of disruption in our lives that extends to other personal relationships, our work and leisure. The yearning and searching associated with bereavement are our responses to the loose ends of caring, unanchored where once there was an object to care. They are responses to ruptures in our personal integrity.

As we grieve, *we reestablish coherence in present living*. We still carry the desires, motivations, dispositions, habits, behaviors, and day-to-day expectations and hopes that once were grounded in the relationships with the deceased. These ties persist as we repeatedly anticipate experiences or initiate actions that make sense only when we can interact in person with the deceased. As we continue to anticipate such interaction, we find ourselves over and over again distressingly "out of sync" with reality. If we cope by persisting in ways that are no longer viable, we live in fantasy, no longer in the present but in the past. In order to relearn ourselves in present reality, we must establish a new pattern of living in which we fill time in different ways and invest ourselves in alternative experiences and activities. As we modify our daily lives, we change the encompassing shape and pattern of those lives. We find our way within, and learn how to be ourselves in, our new present reality.

We Seek New Ways to Complete Our Life Stories

Most of David's past experience outside the family was with Bobby. He played and explored the world with him daily. They dreamed of the future together. Bobby's death occurs in David's formative years, before his unfolding life story supports any firm sense of personal identity. As a major turning point, the death disrupts his early development and no doubt alters its pattern as David incorporates a major loss into his life pattern despite his limited coping capacities. He is not self-consciously aware of its significance, but later he may become so. He struggles against the nightmares that threaten to obliterate all happy memories of Bobby and their play times together. He works to regain equilibrium in, and motivation for, his present life in his family, at school, and with other friends. And he must find hopes for the future that do not include living near Bobby, having him as a best friend next door and at school, and becoming a baseball player with him. His early, and extremely painful, first experience with death will echo as he experiences later losses, forms and values friendships, and parents children of his own and, possibly, as he chooses a career.

Thirty-five years of married life with Earl made Margaret who she was. She built her daily life around him. She looked forward to a new relationship with him in his retirement. Margaret transforms herself remarkably as she works through her ambivalence toward Earl. As she grieves, she comes to view the story of her life and the death in a new light. She still fully appreciates, and vows never to forget, all the good things Earl provided, including shelter, comfort, security, material well-being, home, family, affection and intimacy, companionship, friendship, patience, forgiveness, financial security for her children, and a place in the community. In death, he still provides for her and her family, and she remains ever grateful. But she honestly acknowledges the limits that marriage to Earl placed on her. She finds her past life too confining and her past self too dependent on, and at times controlled by, Earl. She interprets the present as a time to discover her own long-suppressed potential. She no longer defines her future in terms of sharing Earl's retirement years. Instead, she radically revises her hopes and dreams, looks forward to an unprecedented independence and self-reliance, and sees her future as a time to use her new-found potential to know deeper friendships and to contribute to her family and community in new ways. As she realizes how much she is changing and senses the excitement of it, she cautiously looks forward to more unexpected, yet welcome, changes. She knows that having known Earl and having lost him when she did have changed her forever. She realizes that his fortune has made her flourishing possible, and for this, too, she is grateful.

When we are bereaved, *we experience incompleteness in our-selves* as loss disrupts the continuity of our life stories. As we live in and shape our autobiographies, we come to understand ourselves. We experience our lives as having meaning and purpose rooted in histories of past experience, sustained in present living, and projected in expectations and hopes about how our stories will continue to unfold. Bereavement renders incoherent the stories of our lives with those who died and undermines both the self-identity and the sense of meaning and purpose we previously found in those stories. So much of the weaving and reweaving of the webs of our personal integrity then seems irretrievably unraveled. Often, when we are bereaved, we experience our past as too painful to remember, our present life as too distressing and confusing, and many of our expectations, hopes, and dreams as no longer viable. Some of us, like Margaret, become more aware of our own mortality and come to feel responsibility for giving meaning and purpose to the remaining chapters of our autobiographies.

As we grieve, *we struggle to give new sense and direction to the continuing stories of our lives.* We seek new direction, purpose, and meaning as we live our autobiographies. The death of someone close is a pivotal turning point for us and changes forever the narratives of our lives. As we cope, we reconnect with the past, present, and future in senseful ways. We develop new perspectives on, or reinterpret, our past relationship with those who died and the life we built around that relationship; we pursue new meaning and purpose in our present daily living; and we redefine our expectations, hopes, and dreams for the future. As we again find or establish coherence in our lives, we regain our bearings in our own life histories and secure new self-identities. We experience our lives as "making sense" to us again and again "know who we are." In short, we pursue viable ways of going on with our lives.

Because our selves are historical, fluid, and always open to development, none of us finishes becoming a self (shaping a life narrative) until death. So, too, none of us ever really completes relearning in the light of major losses. As we reach other major turning points or incur other losses, we often revise and adjust our accommodation to earlier loss. At each point of revision we may revisit and find new meanings in the earlier loss events, the lives of the deceased, and the lives we lived with them. In turn, how we cope with earlier loss is likely to influence our later coping.

David's story would have been markedly different had his father rather than Bobby died. He would have lost one of the two most

important adults in his life, and the effects on his personal development would have been far more dramatic and decisive. The immediate challenges of relearning his past, present, and future would
have been greater, and at later stages of his development, the absence of his father would have meant far more than the absence of
his six-year-old friend. Limited memories of his father would have
been more difficult to live with, and the ongoing absence of his father would have led to far-reaching differences in his life pattern.
The pain of not having his father to lean on or to model his behavior
would have compounded the echoes of the death at other turning
points or times of loss in his life. And the story would have been
different still, of course, if his mother were to remarry.

Margaret's story well illustrates the challenges and the rewards
of continually reweaving losses into life patterns, self-understandings, and self-identities. We can experience losses as *"tragic
opportunities"*—tragic because our losses are, typically at least, dis-
tressful events that befall us and that we must cope with and opportunities because they allow us to become whole in ways that we
have never been whole before. As we, like Margaret, transform ourselves, we may develop new capacities, realize new meanings, find
new purposes, experience unprecedented flourishing, or achieve
new levels of self-understanding. We may even become more self-
conscious, self-directive, and self-possessed in giving new shape to
our lives and finding new self-confidence and self-esteem. Margaret
realizes all of these possibilities. David, too, may one day find some
such benefits in his experience with loss. The opportunities for realizing these possibilities are reiterated throughout our lifetimes as
we encounter the recurring challenge to reweave the losses into the
stories of our lives. Reminders of our own mortality can provide
powerful inducement to take advantage of such tragic opportunities, as they do in Margaret's case.

We Become Whole Again as Parts of Larger Wholes

David senses that only his parents are safe, and he loses contact with
friends. He also loses temporarily the excitement of beginning
school. He has no developed concept of God or the meaning of life,
though what he overhears adults saying puzzles him. The loss of his
best friend at an early age is likely to color his later thinking about
his place in the greater scheme of things, as will his unspoken fear of
his own mortality. David has yet to experience the richness of meaning and sense of purpose that he can realize as a part of larger wholes.

Perhaps he withdraws into the shelter of his family to reassure himself that the only self-transcending connections he has known aside from those with Bobby still hold. The death shakes his ability to trust any connection beyond the family. His counselor and his parents bring him back to a life pattern typical of a six-year-old boy as he returns to school and picks up with new friendships. Even so, he senses that his friends find him strange, and he is not yet comfortable with them. The death may have long-term consequences for his ability to feel at home in or to join and participate actively in anything larger than himself.

When Mary and the children died, Margaret was alienated from Earl, though she stayed with him. By the time Earl dies she has lost so many of those on whom she has lavished her love and caring that she is tempted to think such devotion is futile. As devastating as her losses are, she never wavers in her faith in God. Yet she wonders whether she can live meaningfully in a seemingly harsh world. Her belief that her remaining years are a gift sustains her. She is no longer dependent as she was with Earl; nor is she entirely devoted to her family or domestic life. She becomes more active, reaches for and accepts help, expands her interests, receives in new ways from others, and makes new contributions. New friendships in the widows' group bring unprecedented satisfactions as at first she receives warm acceptance and support she never knew before and later gives back in kind. Her philanthropic work in cooperation with others on the foundation project brings new wholeness into her life and a greater connection with the larger community. She is especially gratified that in enlisting the help and support of her family in her philanthropy she unites them in a common purpose and fosters new family bonds. Her sense of doing God's work in the process, of making good use of the gift of life, is humbling and rewarding.

When we are bereaved, *we experience ourselves as disconnected from larger wholes* of which we thought ourselves parts. We are deprived of the meaning and purpose provided by the connections within the web of webs. Obviously, we lose the give-and-take with the deceased. Sometimes lines of connection with our fellow survivors strain or break, and we absorb secondary losses. Some of us also lose motivation for work or other creative activities that have helped us to flourish and to sense that we make a difference while we are alive. As we disconnect in these ways, we lose much of what supports our self-image, self-confidence, self-esteem, and individuality. The loss of spiritual place described in Chapter 4 leaves us feeling no longer at home in the world and out of touch with the transcendent purposes of living, however we conceive them. In some instances, we experience ourselves as distant from, or even betrayed by, God.

As we grieve *we recover or find wholeness as parts of larger wholes*. We reconnect with our surviving families and friends and with new persons who enter our lives. We reconnect with the broader community through our work, volunteer, social activist, or other creative activities. And we reconnect with God or the greater powers and larger histories and purposes of the universe, however we may conceive them. As we do so, we combine still viable patterns of give-and-take with new ones in life patterns that support renewed, and possibly quite different, self-images, self-concepts, self-confidence, and self-esteem. Within our connections to our families, friends, and the broader communities we struggle to once again experience ourselves as flourishing, making contributions, being valued, and living with meaning and purpose. Within our connections to God or the greater forces of the universe, we seek such things as acceptance, a sense of belonging, forgiveness, peace, solace, and ultimate meaning and purpose. As we reshape and establish ourselves in connections, we experience ourselves as becoming whole again.

We differ considerably in our ways of making and maintaining connections with others, depending on our individual styles. Our coping varies, for example, with our patterns of independence, interdependence, and dependence in the relationships that remain. Some of us are more active or more passive. We expect different things of others, make different demands, and accept different demands as partners in the reintegration process. Some of us, like Margaret, break with earlier styles as we either transform preexisting relationships or form new ones.

Together We Reshape Our Families and Communities

When Bobby dies, David loses the first and the best friend he ever had. His parents, seeing the effects of Bobby's death on David, begin to act differently, far more protectively, toward him. He is frightened by the glimpses he gets of their anger at Bobby's parents, and he misses the fun he had under their watchful eye in the house and yard next door. He feels ill at ease at school and with his other friends, who don't really know what to make of what has happened to him. They weren't as close to Bobby and have not ever lost their own best friends. David's coping capacities and patterns are just forming, and his parents provide early modeling for these capacities. Their concern about his reaction to Bobby's death and their willingness to bring him to, and cooperate with, his counselor indicate that he will be in some ways well supported by them; their refusal to take him to the funeral and their failure to sense that he might have questions about his experience indicate that in other ways he may not be well supported by them. The exact nature of the legacy of Bobby's death for David's future coping is unpredictable, but his early effectiveness when helped by the counselor is promising.

Margaret strongly identified with the ongoing life of her family, and it pains her to experience the shattering of the well-established family life pattern. Relationships with her surviving children and grandchildren and among them are strained in ways that leave her near despair because few family members are as comfortably at home in the family as they had been. Just when she needs family support, they seem least ready to provide it. Margaret had learned to cope straightforwardly, instinctually, and largely independently in her family of origin, among her peers, and in her family life with Earl. After the deaths, she works to change that no longer effective pattern. She breaks with her own coping precedents and learns a new pattern with the help of her counselor and the widows' group. She becomes more self-reflective and deliberate and far more willing to reach out for and to accept others' support. These changes are themselves a positive legacy of Earl's death. For Margaret, the devastation in her family makes the others relatively unavailable to provide the immediate help and support she needs. When Earl dies, the person on whom she has relied the most through so many years is simply no longer available to comfort her when she needs him most. Many of her friends simply fail her altogether as they turn away in discomfort.

When we are bereaved, *we experience the impacts of loss within our own families and the broader community.* Loss of a member of our families or communities can be represented by the effective removal of the web that represents the life of the deceased from the web of webs that represents these broader social contexts. Loss affects family and community members simultaneously yet in distinctive ways, since connections with the deceased and with fellow survivors differ. The shattered coherence in our present family and community lives corresponds to the shattered coherence in our present individual lives. Disruption and incompleteness within our families and our community narratives correspond to the disruption and incompleteness of our individual narratives. And the breakdown of established connections within our families and communities corresponds to our individual disconnectedness. We suffer as individuals, then, in the broader contexts of collective family and community suffering. As we identify with the ongoing lives of our families and communities, we share in the collective experiences of loss of wholeness in them. These broader impacts define in part the surrounding world context within which we transform our lives through coping with loss.

We become the selves we are in interaction with our social surroundings, beginning with the family in infancy and continuing throughout a lifetime. Our selves are essentially social and interdependent, and we weave our webs of personal integrity within a web of webs that supports and sustains us. *We cope as individuals, then, against a background of social interaction and within a particular social context.* This social context provides historical and personal developmental conditions within which we cope and conditions our progress.

Within the history of the interdependent weaving of the web of personal integrity and in our present living within the web of webs, we learn and are reinforced in the motivations, dispositions, habits, virtues and vices, patterns of emotional response, thought patterns and beliefs, expectations, self-images, self-concepts, self-confidence, self-esteem, self-understanding, and coping capacities that we bring to bear on our experiences of loss. Moreover, the histories and legacies of our previous losses, including but not limited to losses through death, are part of our social histories and legacies. We remember together with others and set precedents for our coping as we grieve alongside and witness others who also grieve. From others we learn patterns of behavior, expression, and interaction in the aftermath of loss, and together we interpret the meanings of what we have all experienced. With others we develop understandings of the possibilities of self-transformation through grieving. In some social contexts patterns can become rigid, and often an inertia develops that leads us to repeat patterns in new loss experiences. We cope under the influence of, and often in the intimate settings of, families, within which myths and legends, norms, ideals, and beliefs, patterns of dependence and autonomy, dominance and deference, support and encouragement, and patterns of give-and-take at times support us as we cope effectively and at other times inhibit or constrain our coping. We also cope within broader social and cultural contexts in which comparable expectations and preexisting patterns color our private experience, our ways of expressing ourselves, and our ways of relearning our worlds.

We often acquire expectations of support from selected others that we bring to our loss experiences. As happened for Margaret, shifts in the availability of others on whom we rely can complicate our coping. Bereavement affects our fellow survivors differently, and some who are normally very supportive and helpful may find themselves devastated. Some who have come through for us before may have grown distant, moved away, or died; still others may simply fail to come through. Such failures of support compound the impacts of loss upon us and compromise our coping effectiveness. Of particular note and poignancy here is the loss of support from the one who has died, whose support might have been forthcoming and welcome in other times of trouble. We cope more effectively if we can find the social support we need, even if at times we do so in quite unexpected or unprecedented places.

Social factors, such as differences in gender, age, economic class, ethnic origin, and culture often decisively influence our individual coping. Others' expectations of us and the support they provide for us as we grieve are similarly socially conditioned. Within the web of webs, the prevailing social conditions for coping vary considerably from one location to another. Some families, for example, acknowledge and support children or the elderly in their grief (as in David's case), while others nearly ignore them. Some families encourage men and women alike to develop and express their emotional selves, while other families sharply differ in their treatment of them. The contrasts between the grieving of Earl and Bill on the one hand and of Margaret and Diane on the other illustrate this point well. Some friends acknowledge men's struggles with loss, while others dismiss them. Bill's struggle in the Rotary Club is an example. Some communities or ethnic groups expect the views and directions of authority figures to prevail. Deference to Earl complicates Margaret's early grieving in this way. Last, members of different economic classes utilize the various available social support services differently. Fortunately, such services are available to and recommended for David and Margaret. These socially reinforced differences in coping strategies sometimes make all the difference in whether we are supported effectively in our grieving.

We cope in social contexts, with others who are mourning the loss of the same person. We reweave the web of our daily lives, reshape our autobiographies, and establish connection interdependently with larger wholes. This can comfort or reassure us that we do not grieve in isolation. However, we are also constrained by our interdependence. We simply do not entirely control the emerging results of coping. We emerge as transformed selves as the result of the combination and interaction of several individuals' coping. The enacted decisions of one person who addresses particular tasks both affect and provide the context for the decisions of others. None of us can foresee the results of our coping because none of us can predict the decisions, actions, and reactions of others that shape the new world within which each of us finds a new identity. The shape of our new lives within our families and communities is not entirely within our individual control. We share responsibility for redefining family and community life that in turn conditions our individual possibilities.

This social interdependence and the historically fluid nature of our selves partially define the mystery of our individual lives. As we transform ourselves in social contexts, the results of our coping are unforeseeable, and our coping is never finished. While addressing particular tasks as we relearn our worlds is like solving problems, the cumulative effect of our addressing those tasks is quite different. Overcoming suffering and finding new wholeness in our lives, like any process of personal development, so depend on other's influences and contributions that they are never completed, and ever mysterious.

We jointly change the fabric of social interaction and the life, flourishing, and realization of meaning sustained within that fabric. We reweave the web of webs together. At times, what any one of us wants most fervently will simply not come to pass. Margaret hopes for a closeness with her daughters and daughters-in-law like that she finds in the widows' group, but her hopes are only partially realized. This can be frustrating or worse. On the other hand, our combined efforts can yield unprecedented and welcome new patterns and experiences. Coping with others changes not only personal history but also shared history. Just as we come to new ways of being ourselves as individuals, so we in community with others find and create new ways of being together. Families and communities transform themselves as they grieve together. These efforts, in turn, support or limit our individual abilities to flourish and to find personal narratives meaningful. As we join in reweaving the web of webs, some of us experience ourselves as parts of self-transcending wholes. This is Margaret's experience as she enlists family members' assistance in her philanthropy.

Advantages of the Idea of Relearning Our Selves

It is common to conceive of our selves as so many atoms afloat in social space. Our personal integrity, on this metaphor, is a matter quite independent of our worldly entanglements. We are thought of as self-contained, impenetrable, and isolated in our individuality and independence. When this metaphor is taken seriously, relationships and involvements in the world are conceived as matters external to our integrity. Relationships have nothing to do with either individual personal integrity or personal identity, both of which supposedly develop and are sustained within the atoms themselves and not by the interactions among them. Love, for example, becomes a matter of attraction between atoms, proximate location of mutually attracted atoms, and perhaps harmonious vibrations between them. But the metaphor requires that as selves in our relationships we remain unchanged. The death of another is seen as nothing more than the disappearance of a completely independent entity, another social atom, that hovered nearby for a time. Even if the attraction between us was strong and if as paired atoms we were vibrating on the same wavelength in a social groove, the mere disappearance would not affect matters internal to the one of us left vibrating alone. Major bereavements would thus leave the integrity and the identity of our selves unaffected. I believe such imagery overemphasizes our independence while utterly failing to capture anything of our permeability or interdependence. It reflects nothing of the contributions to our personal development and the transformation over time that our relationships and involvements in the world entail.

The Idea Provides General Understanding

The web metaphor has considerable advantage over such atomistic thinking because it supports more adequate understanding of our selves and our personal development prior to bereavement. It captures much of the character of the development of our self-images, self-concepts, self-confidence, self-esteem, personal integrity, and personal identities as they emerge in our unfolding personal histories and within broad social contexts. It captures the social, permeable, and interdependent character of our selves and the influence of the patterns of caring involvement in the world that determine who we are.

The web metaphor illuminates the vulnerability of our selves to

suffering and to loss of wholeness in bereavement. It supports understanding of how in bereavement we experience the loss of wholeness embodied in the coherence of our present life patterns, the
integrity of our life stories, and our connections with larger wholes.
It captures the searing penetration of our selves that we so frequently experience when someone we care about dies. Where there is
inattention to such a potential for suffering, our suffering is likely
to be compounded unnecessarily. Though conceptual clarity will
not make our human vulnerability any the less real, it can ground
an understanding (including a self-understanding) of that suffering
that in itself is a part of a humane response to it.

We far too often think of ourselves as self-contained, impenetrable, and isolated in our integrity and identity. Such thinking is
actively encouraged by the idealization of rugged individualism and
independence. If we accept the atomistic ways of thinking of ourselves, we do not expect the shattering impacts of loss. Our relationships can and do mean a great deal to most of us, but few of us
appreciate how the connectedness that such relationships afford is
integral to the unique persons we are. Surprise at the nature, intensity, and pervasiveness of the effects of loss often unsettles us. Loss
not only validates the thinking captured in the web metaphor but
in some instances is the occasion for a shift in self-understanding.
Where no such shift occurs, many of us doubt ourselves and begin
to wonder whether we are losing touch with reality. The inadequacy of our understanding of our own shattered selves obscures the
reality of how much our relationships meant. This lack reflects the
inadequacies of the culturally dominant atomistic ways of thinking
of our selves. We do not casually fail to acknowledge an obvious
and fundamental dimension of our human nature and vulnerability;
rather, a failure in the predominant way of thinking blocks recognition of that nature and vulnerability.

Finally, the web metaphor supports our understanding of our
coping with loss as a multifaceted struggle toward wholeness in our
present life patterns, ongoing autobiographies, and connections
with larger wholes. The metaphor of reweaving the web of the self
captures each of the relieving, restorative, and transformative functions of our coping. Moreover, imagining individual webs within
the broader social and historical context of the web of webs captures the ways our coping is built on, supported within, and conditioned by our social interactions and by the ongoing histories of the
larger communities of which we are parts.

The Idea Promotes Respect for Individuality

The web metaphor for personal integrity and the social, permeable, and interdependent nature of our selves well captures both the sources of our uniqueness and the uniqueness of our experiences of loss. The image is as complex, subtle, and nuanced as we are as individuals. No two of our selves are identical. No two of us inhabit the same social and historical contexts. No two of us have the same habits, dispositions, motivations, virtues and vices, patterns of emotional response, thought patterns and beliefs, expectations, hopes and aspirations, self-images, self-concepts, self-confidence, self-esteem, self-understanding, and coping capacities. No two of us live the same personal histories, flourish in identical ways, or realize the same meanings and purposes. No two of us are vulnerable to, or experience, identical impacts of losses or address identical tasks as we cope with them. No two of us are supported and sustained, or constrained and inhibited, in identical ways within identical social and historical circumstances. No two of us grieve together with the same fellow survivors or play identical roles in reconstituting the social fabric and redefining the histories of our families and larger communities. The web metaphor, but not the atomistic alternative, captures and illuminates all of these aspects of our uniqueness as selves, our vulnerability to suffering, and our coping with loss.

The Idea Addresses Our Helplessness

The web metaphor also serves as a basis for understanding our helplessness and what is required if we are to overcome it. It illuminates the often paralyzing effects of the suffering that bereavement entails. It fosters understanding of the challenges of coping, the direction for effectively addressing them, and the specific tasks of self-reintegration and self-transformation that can move our grieving forward. As it accounts for the surprise and self-doubt that often accompany bereavement, it supports overcoming their often crippling effects.

Where atomistic concepts of self prevail, many who suffer only reluctantly seek help from others in the mistaken belief that their problems are entirely internal. As the web metaphor shows how our selves are socially constructed and interdependent and how our coping is socially conditioned and supported, it motivates us to recognize the value (and at times the near necessity) of reaching out to others. It helps us to overcome our expectations of self-reliance when they inhibit our progress. It moves us to take an active role in the joint effort to reconstruct the social fabric and to redefine our family and community histories in the aftermath of loss.

The Idea Provides Guidance for Caregivers

A tendency to fight feelings of tenderness and compassion with toughness often inhibits those of us who are in the thrall of atomistic thinking from offering help. This tendency overemphasizes self-reliance, insists that we take care of ourselves, and makes others suspicious of those of us who cannot or will not do so. These unfortunate consequences of atomistic thinking further isolate those of us who suffer in bereavement just when we most need connection with others.

In contrast, the web metaphor helps define specific approaches that we as caregivers can use to support and comfort those who suffer. It recognizes that grieving persons transform themselves within social contexts that either hinder or support them. As caregivers we can help the bereaved to understand that their self-doubt and their experience of themselves as shattered by the loss are normal. We can help them recognize that their suffering is a function of their loss of wholeness and help them find the motivation to overcome the shattering effects of loss and to struggle toward renewed wholeness.

As caregivers, *we can support others as they struggle to establish coherence in present living* by establishing a new pattern of desires, motivations, dispositions, habits, behaviors, and hopes and expectations that is congruent with a reality where the deceased is absent. We can offer understanding and reassurance that the persistence of the old ways is normal. We can comfort and support the bereaved as they feel and express their distress and anguish over the incompatibility of lingering patterns and current reality. We can offer them our patience, encouragement, and support as they identify and let go of what is no longer viable and rebuild daily routines that restore still viable elements of the old and add new ones. As we do so, we help those who grieve to find a new equilibrium in present living.

As caregivers, *we can help the bereaved to find new direction, purpose, and meaning in their life stories.* We can help them to reconnect with their past, present, and future in meaningful ways. We can offer comfort and support as they feel and express their distress and anguish over the disruption in their life stories. We can support them as they review, seek new perspectives on, and reinterpret past events, the past relationship with the deceased, and the life built around it. We can encourage and support them as they recover still viable purposes and meanings in present living and seek new ones. And we can offer our patience, encouragement, and support as they revive still viable expectations, hopes, and dreams and define new ones. As we do so, we help those who grieve to find themselves once again at home in life stories that make sense to them.

As caregivers, *we can help the bereaved to find meaningful connection to larger wholes.* We can offer comfort and support as they feel and express the distress and anguish over broken connections. We can help them to establish new patterns of give-and-take that at least provide a basis for flourishing that they experience as comparable in value to the one they had enjoyed prior to the death and that enable them to revive satisfactory self-images, self-concepts, self-confidence and self-esteem. We can give reassurance as they doubt whether they themselves or what they do matter. We can encourage and support them as they rebuild still viable connections to family, friends, and the broader community. We can offer guidance when solicited and support them as they explore connections with God or the greater forces of the universe, struggle to recover their sense of spiritual place, and seek acceptance, forgiveness, peace, consolation, and ultimate meaning and purpose based in faith or conviction. And we can encourage and support them as they seek to overcome past dependence or passivity in relationships, establish new relationships with others, seek and undertake new avenues for giving or contributing, or pursue new hopes, aspirations, meanings, or purposes along the lines of connection in their lives. As we do so, we help them again to experience themselves as parts of meaningful wholes.

As it shows the ways our coping is socially interdependent, the understanding rooted in the web metaphor enables us as caregivers to appreciate how our compassion, empathy, and supportive efforts contribute to the self-transformation of those who grieve along renewed or new lines of connection with us, the caregivers. And it promotes in us as caregivers a sense of community and of our shared responsibility with those who grieve to reweave the social fabric and to author together the next chapters of our community narratives.

In all of these ways, the web metaphor supports understanding of the common humanity shared by us and our caregivers and experienced in the intricate and delicate interweavings of human relationships. It also promotes respect for the uniqueness of our selves as we

embody unprecedented, fragile, and irreplaceable patterns of caring
and connection in distinctive social circumstances.

Notes

1. The discussion of the paralyzing emotion grief in Chapter 2 illustrates this aspect of suffering.

2. I came to fully appreciate this insight in conversation with Phyllis
Silverman as she told of how survivors of the Holocaust have learned to
carry their sorrows.

3. Recall the discussion in Chapter 3 of individual vulnerabilities of
these kinds.

6

Relearning Our Relationships
with the Deceased:
Grief, Love, and Separation

Kathryn's Story

When Mark dies from an inoperable brain tumor at age thirty-eight, his wife, Kathryn, is prepared for the inevitable but devastated nevertheless. The world, it seems, has dealt her and their two children, Josh and Sarah, not to mention Mark, a cruel blow. She had tasted powerlessness as Mark's illness ran its inevitable and punishing course. However, neither she nor Mark was ever inclined to allow events to control or overwhelm them, no matter how unpredictable and seemingly arbitrary they might be. Having married Mark after receiving her M.S. in nursing at age twenty-three, Kathryn had enjoyed a successful career for the first ten years of their marriage before acceding to the demands of her "biological clock," choosing to have the children and planning to return to her career only when they were in school.

Mark lived nearly a year after the tumor was discovered. Neither he nor Kathryn had any choice about the unrelenting course of the growth of the tumor and its predicted outcome. Both resolved to do all they could, both for themselves and for the children, as they anticipated the profound changes to come in their lives. They prepared

The thinking in the chapter is an elaboration and refinement of that found in my "Grief, Love and Separation," in *Death: Completion and Discovery* (Hartford: Forum for Death Education and Counseling, 1987).

a living will in anticipation of complications in the end stages of his illness, planned his funeral, and revised their wills sooner than either found comfortable. They told Josh and Sarah what was happening, answered their questions patiently, provided much comfort and support, and assured them that they would be well taken care of when Daddy died. They had managed to save money before the children arrived, and insurance would carry Kathryn until the children were in school and provide a cushion of additional savings should she return to her career or pursue advanced training.

Mark and Kathryn talked often of her life after Mark's death, candidly expressed their hopes and fears, and provided each other what comfort they could. Mark always admired Kathryn's ambition and abilities and consistently supported her. He wholeheartedly encouraged her to pursue her career interests after his death and to consider seeking specialized advanced training. A career in nursing administration appeared well within her reach. Both were sad that Mark would not be by her side through the struggles to come and to share in any future successes.

Mark startled Kathryn when he acknowledged that she might one day choose to remarry and sincerely encouraged her to consider doing so. He wrote her a letter that expressed concerns about Josh and Sarah's growing up without a father and Kathryn's living without a companion. He recognized that she would grieve following his death, but he urged her not to allow herself to be consumed by the grief. He said he could die more peacefully if he knew she was determined to meet the challenges of grieving and to move beyond them to find happiness despite his death. Because he loved her, he wanted her to become all she could be and to flourish in life with their children, in her career, and with a life's companion, if she chose to have one. He went so far as to ask her to promise that she would not allow grief to overcome her, to defeat her. Kathryn responded in disbelief at his courage. She doubted she would hurry to find a future companion, but she thanked Mark for his generous love.

Mark made it clear that he feared being forgotten, and Kathryn assured him that that was not possible for her. His greatest fear, however, was that Josh and Sarah might forget, or that they would have only hazy memories of a figure frozen in photographs. He longed so to be a part of their lives as they lived their childhood years and grew to adulthood. Painful as it was to leave Kathryn, it was even more difficult to say good-bye to the children without knowing them in the fullness of their lives.

Mark's condition worsened in the early fall, and it became clear that he probably would not see another Christmas. Kathryn foresaw an outpouring of concern for her and for the children at the holiday season as the usual flood of holiday cards and letters came in. She anticipated that the correspondence might include remembrances of Mark. She secretly wrote a letter addressed to everyone on their extensive Christmas list and explained that Mark was dying and unlikely to see the holidays. She asked everyone to write early and to recount stories and memories of Mark that could be collected and shared with him before he died. The response overwhelmed her and warmed her heart. Nearly one hundred pieces came from relatives and friends across the country, many including extensive memories, stories of Mark previously unknown to her, photographs, and expressions of concern and affection for Mark and the family. As Mark's condition worsened, but while he was lucid and energetic, she put everything in scrapbooks, presented them to Mark, and spent three wonderful evenings with him alternately reading and commenting on what they received, remembering together, crying and holding each other close, and sharing with the children what they seemed interested in and capable of understanding. Mark told her it was the most wonderful gift he ever received. They had never felt closer.

Though she anticipated Mark's death, Kathryn did not anticipate how she would miss him everywhere. She now notices his absence in every corner of her home and life. She longs for him intensely. She visits his grave often and fingers her wedding ring repeatedly each day. Yet she soon sees the hazards of dwelling in her clearly futile and frustrating longing for Mark's return. She remembers his admonitions and her promise not to be consumed with grief for him and to get on with her life. She feels encouraged by Mark and well supported by him as she grieves.

Kathryn takes comfort in talking to Mark in his absence, at the cemetery, while alone as she fingers her ring, as she prepares for the day before the mirror, and as she closes the day in prayer. As she adapts her daily routine and the pattern of her life, she finds comfort in his presence in memory and inspiration to get on with living and caring for Josh and Sarah. She enjoys "remember-when" sessions with them. As she makes important decisions about her own and their lives, she regularly engages in internal dialogue with Mark, seeking his advice and counsel while no more giving him the final say than she had while he was alive. Instead, she senses his sentiments and the course he might have tried to persuade her to follow, and she takes his "advice" into account in settling her own mind on the matter.

Kathryn treasures the years she spent with Mark and realizes that they cannot be taken away from her. They touched her deeply, changed her profoundly, filled her with memories, provided resources to cope with adversity and meet challenges head on and confidently, left her with two wonderful children, and filled her with a zest for living; no doubt, they still influence and inspire her in ways she is only beginning to understand. Once beyond the pain of her seemingly unrelenting longing, she sees that the meaning of the years with Mark is not canceled. She has a loving legacy to hold to herself, to allow to shape ensuing years of her life as she chooses, and to share with Josh and Sarah.

Each year, during the holidays and on Mark's birthday, Kathryn takes out the scrapbooks of remembrances of Mark and finds new inspiration. She shares the materials selectively with Josh and Sarah. It gratifies her that each year they have new questions about their father and seem to be getting to know him better. She remembers Mark's concern that he not be forgotten by the children or merely remembered as a figure frozen in a photograph, and the intensity of the children's interest touches her. Her confidence grows that Mark is a living presence in their lives as she sees them so often grasping something new in the stories and remembrances, as they occasionally refer to him in day-to-day life, and as they grow in ways that would have pleased Mark and that reflect something of his influence.

Kathryn returns for advanced training in nursing administration and later joins a nursing faculty. While she does so primarily for herself and the children, she is grateful to Mark for encouraging her career development and for his continuing inspiration to be all she can be. When she is most discouraged about the burdens of raising their children and continuing her studies, she realizes that her perseverance derives in part from his influence. She dedicates her professional efforts to Mark's memory.

Five years after Mark's death, Kathryn remarries. Jim is also widowed, but he is childless. Jim and Kathryn appreciate the memories and legacies each brings from the previous marriage, as well as the continuing burden of pain. They hear each other's stories and those of their dead spouses, acknowledge the sadness they share, and eventually feel grateful that the other was so touched and shaped by the earlier marriage. Both are sensitive to the need to build a new relationship on its own terms while respecting the legacies of the previous marriages and their attendant emotional needs. They agree that much remembering of the earlier marriages can be done privately or with family or friends who knew their first spouses. When either experiences pain in memory or encounters a new challenge in grieving, the other provides comfort as requested and needed. Jim is especially sensitive to Josh's and Sarah's needs to continue to allow their father a place in their lives. He encourages Kathryn to continue the holiday and birthday traditions she had established before remarrying, though he prefers not to be present. While he comes to love the children as if they were his own, he always respects their needs to be Mark's children. Kathryn senses Jim's pain in this and respects his courage in not insisting on closer ties.

Colleen's Story

Colleen was estranged from her daughter Sheila since her late teens. Colleen was smothering, controlling, and protective after her divorce from Jack, Sheila's father. Sheila resisted, argued bitterly with her mother during her last years of high school, used alcohol (like her father) to escape pain and to rebel against her mother, and spent as little time at home as she could get away with. She welcomed the chance to use the money (provided for the purpose when the divorce was settled) to escape to college in another state. She stopped answering her mother's letters and phone calls. Colleen, exasperated and fearing she would provoke her daughter further, stopped trying to control her life and eventually concluded that Sheila needed most to be completely on her own. She hoped that Sheila one day would understand her mother's difficulties after the divorce, her pain when Sheila left for college, and her wish for only the best in life for Sheila, even if it meant permanent estrangement. Though she wished that reconciliation were possible, Colleen doubted she would hear from Sheila again.

Sheila graduated from college and began a life on her own with a publishing company in the same major West Coast city where she went to school. She began to enjoy considerable success, and she made friends easily. Her lifestyle supported and encouraged her continued use of alcohol, but she considered herself only a "social drinker." She never married, and, though she dated extensively, she had no companion. Having witnessed her parents' marriage, she hesitated about making commitments that might lead to marriage. When she was twenty-seven, she began on a downward spiral with depressive illness. The combination of the illness and her growing abuse of alcohol led eventually to her suicide.

Remarkably, and much to Colleen's relief, Sheila called her

mother in the middle of her twenty-eighth year with a desire to re-connect. They began hesitatingly, with weekly phone calls and an exchange of letters. Colleen informed her mother of the positive developments in her life and kept the dark side to herself, though she confided to two close friends that it was fear of that dark side that had moved her to contact her mother. Colleen traveled to the Coast for a holiday visit only three months before Sheila took an overdose of antidepressant medication with a large vodka chaser. In conversations and on her visit, Colleen did not detect Sheila's depressive illness through Sheila's efforts to hide it from her. She did not see the suicide coming.

Sheila wrote no suicide note, leaving her friends and family with the mystery of her motives. Each searches his or her soul for understanding of the tragic action, and each struggles to reconcile a love for her with hatred for what she did. The sudden and unexpected disruption in their lives embarrasses some who are uncomfortable with the social stigma of suicide. Jack, with drink in hand, tells Colleen at the wake that he has no doubt that Colleen's failures as a mother eventually drove Sheila to kill herself. Though she defends herself against the cruelty of his remarks, Colleen struggles internally with her guilt and anguish over her inability to reach Sheila during the difficult years after the divorce. Some resent the apparent selfishness of Sheila's act, and still others insist that the death was accidental. The funeral period is filled with awkward silences as few are comfortable in talking about the life that ended so tragically. Preoccupation with the events leading to the death submerges people's ability to remember Sheila as she lived.

Colleen alone wants to learn more about Sheila's life. She wants to recover the lost years and to know her daughter better. She finds Sheila's college yearbooks and other personal effects helpful but too sketchy. She decides to go to the Coast to find as many as possible of the people Sheila knew and spent time with at work and socially. The life now ended is simply too precious to forget, and she wants to know and understand better how Sheila lived in the years they were estranged, what her friends found attractive in her, and what she seemed to care most about in life. While some of the people she contacts won't speak with her, many are generous with their time and memories. Some show her photos of Sheila with them, and she asks for reprints. She vows to return again later to revisit those who say they would welcome her return and to find others who are not available when she first visits. She keeps a journal record of the conversations and fills in the missing pages of the story of Sheila's life as she builds a memory book.

Family and friends express skepticism about Colleen's activities, doubting that it is "good for her" to be so "preoccupied" or "obsessed" with Sheila. Still, she persists and finds the activity one of the most meaningful things she has ever done. It feels neither preoccupying nor obsessive to her, though it is greatly satisfying. She regrets terribly that reconciliation with Sheila did not begin sooner, and she longs for the renewed contact that she cannot now sustain. The interviewing and journal keeping seem to her far more healthy than either maintaining silence about Sheila as if she had never lived (as some seem to want her to do) or pining for her impossible return. She plans only one or two more visits to the West Coast in the next year and doubts that she will return thereafter. She carries on otherwise with her daily routine, returns comfortably to work, and resumes a life pattern nearly identical to the one she had known prior to Sheila's death.

Colleen struggles mightily with issues of guilt, anger, forgiveness, and self-forgiveness. She takes some small comfort as she learns through two of her interviews that Sheila recontacted her out of fear of the dark side of her life. She strives to separate her abiding love for Sheila from her anger at Sheila's rebellion and her hatred of her suicide. Recovery of the missing details of the story of Sheila's life helps her sustain her love for her daughter despite her tragic, self-inflicted death. She is saddened as she learns more of Sheila's depression. But she is also surprised and gratified to learn how much Sheila resembled her in caring about such things as literature, the theater, and the environment. Learning more about Sheila's depressive illness and her struggles with alcohol reassures her that Jack's accusation is false, though she wonders if things might have been different if she hadn't been so desperately smothering after the divorce. She wants to understand her daughter better and herself in relation to her. If she made mistakes, and she fears she did, she is determined to learn from them. She struggles to forgive herself for not being there for a daughter who perhaps needed her more than she knew or could comfortably admit. Learning more of the story of Sheila's life promotes her own self-understanding and supports her reevaluation of the meaning of her own life. She is confident that the journal of remembrances and details of Sheila's life will provide a basis for future reflections when she can understand more than she now does.

Sheila's death challenges Colleen spiritually. Her traditional religious background included strong admonitions against suicide, which was viewed as unforgivable, yet she wants very much to forgive Sheila and to believe that she rests safely in the arms of a loving God. As she prays, she prays for Sheila's soul, asks God to help her to understand her grief and the meaning of life, asks Sheila for forgiveness of her "failings" as a mother, expresses gratitude for knowing Sheila during her short life and for what she continues to learn about and from her, and hopes for a reunion in a life to come. Colleen confides with her priest about these spiritual matters as she returns to a more active life in the church. She finds a comfort there that neither friends nor family can provide.

What We Lose, and What We Do Not Lose, When Someone Dies

Writing of his own grief after the death of his beloved wife, C. S. Lewis observed:

> And then one or other dies. And we think of this as love cut short; like a dance stopped in mid-career or a flower with its head unluckily snapped off—something truncated and therefore, lacking its due shape. I wonder. If, as I can't help suspecting, the dead also feel the pains of separation . . . , then for both lovers, and for all pairs of lovers without exception, bereavement is a universal and integral part of our experience of love. It follows marriage as normally as marriage follows courtship or as autumn follows summer. It is not a truncation of the process but one of its phases; not the interruption of the dance, but the next figure.[1]

This eloquent metaphor is a moving expression of how we relearn our relationships with those who die. Lewis's metaphor suggests at least the following: Our loving relationships are dynamic and flowing. When we care about, or love, another person, our attachment resembles the gentle embrace of dancers moving freely together. Something akin to the sensitivity and responsiveness to the unfolding subjectivity of the dance partner is intrinsic to our caring about, and loving, each other. Death does not end our caring or our loving but is compatible with our continuing and transforming our care and our love. As we grieve we struggle to learn the next figures of the dance and to find a meaningful way to continue caring about, and loving, the absent person even as our lives are transformed by our losses. As we grieve, we learn to love in separation.

A closer look at precisely what we do and do not lose of our relationships with the deceased clarifies the variety of challenges we face as we relearn those relationships. Principally, and most obviously, we lose the continuing presence of those we care about and love. This is by no means a simple thing. We also lose the security and the coherence in our lives that were rooted in our expectation that those who died would continue to live. We lose any of the meaning and purpose in our lives that are rooted in our hopes and dreams for future life with the deceased by our sides. We do not lose any of the time lived with the deceased prior to the death. We lose none of what was given to us in our relationships. The meanings of the lives now ended are not canceled; as survivors, we can still incorporate the inspiration and influence of those who have died into our own lives. Our wholeness is affected in many ways by loss. As we grieve, what is lost and what is not defines the impact of loss and the challenges we must address as we grieve.[2]

First, we feel the loss of the other's presence most acutely in our daily lives. Where the everyday lives of the deceased were intimately interwoven with the webs of our lives, as was the case with Mark and Kathryn, there is virtually no moment of our daily living when we fail to notice the absence of the person who had died. No matter how vivid our memories, not seeing those we care about and love, not hearing, not touching or holding, not sharing laughter or tears, not conversing, not deciding together, not greeting or ending the day togehter, even not arguing in person render our memories painfully pale. Our longing for the return of the living presence of the deceased can be downright visceral. Where the everyday life of the deceased was not as intimately interwoven into the webs of our lives, as with Sheila and Colleen, the places and occasions where we feel the lack of presence are usually fewer, though our experiences may be as intense. Colleen feels this lack poignantly as she regrets the lost opportunities in the years of estrangement.

No one should ever underestimate the pain of the loss of a deceased person's presence, no matter the nature of the relationship prior to their death. Orientation through our senses and physical interaction constitutes the primal, biological root of our bonds and attachments. We must overcome, or carry, the pain of such loss. Though our anguish may moderate as we learn to love the deceased in their absence, we will likely experience it still, and it may never vanish. If we are to make the transition to a new relationship with the deceased, we need to move from dwelling in the pain of longing for their presence to enduring and carrying that pain as we adopt a new life pattern that includes our more constructively caring about the deceased in their absence. When we feel the pain and anguish of longing for the deceased most intensely, our pain and anguish themselves may interfere with how well we remember the deceased. When our pain moderates, we may more fully remember and appreciate those who have died. C. S. Lewis captured well this aspect of the transition when he wrote:

> And suddenly at the very moment when, so far, I mourned H. least, I remembered her best. Indeed it was something (almost) better than memory; an instantaneous, unanswerable impression. To say it was like a meeting would be going too far. Yet there was that in it which tempts one to use those words. It was as if the lifting of the sorrow removed a barrier.[3]

In addition to the presence in itself, we lose all of the diverse aspects of day-to-day living that depended on the presence of those who have died. Much of the taken-for-granted in Kathryn's life is no longer viable to the extent that it required Mark's presence. For Colleen, death extinguishes abruptly her recently recovered expectations of a fuller reconciliation with Sheila. Like Kathryn and Colleen, we no longer encounter in the flesh familiar and customary stimuli to emotion, thought, and action. Our daily lives become much more unpredictable. Mundane hopes that have carried us from day to day (for example, the hope to meet for lunch tomorrow or to retire quietly together tonight) are no longer supportable. Neither Mark nor Sheila, nor those we have lost, any longer approach or are approachable in the usual ways with suggestions, requests, or demands; aspects of our selves that were anchored in the relationships with those who died are less readily available to us because they are absent. Consequently, we experience ourselves as less at home in present living. Finally and ironically, some of us, like Kathryn, lose the support in coping with loss that those we love, like Mark, would have provided if they were still present. Correspondingly, but quite differently, for some of us our lingering unfinished business with the deceased, like that between Colleen and Sheila, leaves us without the opportunity to work through important issues with those we have cared about and loved in person.

We lose the presence of central characters in the ongoing stories of our lives. Mark's and Sheila's deaths disrupt Kathryn's and Colleen's autobiographies as they lose their companionship in their lives. When we lose, as they have, we must extinguish and relinquish all expectations of a continued interweaving of our lives with the ongoing lives of those who have died. Strictly speaking, we, like Kathryn and Colleen, never had, and therefore really do not lose, years in the future with those who have died, though we fully expected to have them. As we experience it, however, such is the power of the taken-for-granted in our lives that we often experience the loss of expectations as if it were a deprivation of years together that were fully ours. This loss of our expectations for the future often entails loss of our long-term hopes and dreams and the sense of purpose and meaning in living that we found in them. Kathryn must renew or redefine virtually every aspect of her life story, since her hopes and dreams were so intimately and thoroughly interwoven with the expectation that Mark would be with her in the years to come. Colleen must find the means to make peace with Sheila even though her hopes for fuller reconciliation are dashed. Like Kathryn and Colleen, we must discern the changes in the possibilities now before us in our irrevocably altered life circumstances. We must develop new expectations of ourselves and others and begin to live without those we have lost. We need not abandon all of our expectations, hopes, and dreams, but we will experience even those that we retain differently as we realize them. Like Kathryn and Colleen, we must, in effect, redefine who we are now that those we cared about and loved have died.

We do not lose the years we have lived with the deceased. Like Kathryn's and Colleen's years with Mark and Sheila, our years with those who have died are forever parts of our personal histories. As each of us, like Kathryn and Colleen, redefines and reshapes our own life history in the light of the death, each of us carries the legacy of our relationship with the deceased as at least background to all of our subsequent experience. The consequences of interweaving our lives with those who have left us are still ours, including unresolved problems, memories, influences, and inspirations. Kathryn and Colleen must reintegrate these legacies into their life stories as they remain indelibly touched by Mark and Sheila. So must we all.

We lose our usual ways of connecting with those who have died. Like Kathryn and Colleen, we experience major disruptions in all of our important connections with those, like Mark and Sheila, who have died. Longing for their return is to no avail, and being connected to them in their presence is no longer possible for us. Like Kathryn and Colleen, however, few of us are ready to relinquish all of our ties to the deceased. Though they have died, our love remains strong. As we grieve, we must make a transition from caring about another who is present (most often in a loving way but not necessarily so) to caring about another who is now absent. (This challenge and the ways in which we cope with it are treated later in this chapter.) Like Kathryn and Colleen, we can blend our continued, albeit transformed, caring about and loving of those who have died into the broader pattern of our connections with self-transcending wholes. Kathryn anticipates and addresses the possible complications in a new marital relationship with Jim and gives exploring the meanings of Mark's life a central place in her life with Josh and Sarah. Colleen struggles to redefine her relationship with God and addresses complications in her relationships with fellow survivors who are uncomfortable with her inquiries about Sheila's life.

Let Go We Must, But Not Entirely

We need not break our bonds with the deceased but instead redefine the nature of those bonds and their places in our lives. Rather than challenging us to separate from the dead, their deaths challenge us to maintain meaningful connection and to integrate redefined relationships in our necessarily new life patterns.

We can continue to embrace those who die in their absence. How is it even conceivable that we can continue a dance of love with someone in his or her absence? C. S. Lewis continued the metaphor that I quoted earlier:

> We are "taken out of ourselves" by the loved one while she is here. Then comes the tragic figure of the dance in which we must learn to be still taken out of ourselves though the bodily presence is withdrawn, to love the very Her, and not fall back to loving our past, or our memory, or our sorrow, or our relief from sorrow, or our own love.[4]

Here Lewis urges that we continue to love the very person of the one who died, experienced not as something fixed in time or memory but as someone who retains the power to move us even as we survive him or her. To be sure, it is through our memories and sorrow that we retain access to the very person of the ones we have cared about and loved. However, it is neither our memory nor our sorrow that we care about and love but rather the person we remember in sorrow. Both Mark and Sheila retain the power to touch and influence Kathryn and Colleen, as do so many in our own lives even after they have gone from us.

If it is the person remembered whom we embrace still, what is the nature of our embrace? How can it be a loving embrace? In order to answer, it is necessary to explore the nature of caring and loving attachment, to understand what it is for us to "have" another in a loving relationship. Here, I believe we can learn from Alan Watts:

[T]he greater part of human activity is designed to make permanent those experiences and joys which are only lovable because they are changing. Music is a delight because of its rhythm and flow. Yet the moment you arrest the flow and prolong a note or chord beyond its time, the rhythm is destroyed. . . .[5]

You cannot understand life and its mysteries as long as you try to grasp it. Indeed, you cannot grasp it, just as you cannot walk off with a river in a bucket. If you try to capture running water in a bucket, it is clear that you do not understand it and that you will always be disappointed, for in the bucket the water does not run. To "have" running water you must let go of it and let it run.[6]

Mark, Sheila, and the others in our own lives are ever-changing, dynamic, and flowing like the music or the river. Our loving them in their own right as persons is incompatible with the rigidity and the desperate clinging of a possessiveness based on the illusion of permanence. Our loving instead is like the gentle embrace of partners in a dance. Rather than a way of having something, our loving becomes a way of being with and responding to the rhythm of the lives of the others, a way of being with them through harmony and discord alike. We must be both passive and active, receptive and responsive, as we allow both for their free movement and our spontaneous replies. The only way we can "have" others in such love is for us to let go, to allow them to be other than us or ours. We marvel at the depth and profundity of their independent reality as centers of experience and are moved to respond. Trust in the dynamics of the exchange is not to be confused with the false security of believing we have what we cannot in fact possess, that is, the independent reality of the others in our lives. The only security is that of commitment, its constancy, and of our pledge to stay the course through a loving exchange, person to person.

As we learn to love in this way, we learn to let go and let be. We learn a distinctive form of attachment in separation in which we and those we love are bound by our caring and our mutual involvement, yet retain our own independent reality and develop and flourish in our separateness. Some of us learn these lessons prior to death, as Mark and Kathryn did. Some of us learn them only after our loved one's death, when the reality of not having the one we love comes crashing in. The deeper truth is that we never had the person as a possession even when he or she was alive. Sheila's rebellion clearly derives from her insistence on maintaining her individuality, which Colleen in her smothering failed to recognize. Only late in Sheila's life did Colleen begin to learn about the letting go required to love Sheila as a person in her own right. She continues to learn this lesson after Sheila's death.

Parting is compatible with the continuation of a dance. Some of the finest dance figures are danced in separation as the dancers sustain their connection by their attention and response. We can sustain our connection to those we care about and love even when they are dead. C. S. Lewis wrote:

> All reality is iconoclastic. The earthly beloved, even in this life, incessantly triumphs over your mere idea of her. And you want her to; you want her with all her resistances, all her faults, all her unexpectedness. That is, in her foursquare and independent reality. And this, not any image or memory, is what we are to love still, after she is dead.[7]

Our loving embrace of the dead in their absence is continuous with our loving them when they are present. While our movements of loving exchange change after their death, they do not differ in kind. They can be dynamic and life-affirming.

We need not let go entirely of those who die to avoid becoming obsessive or morbid. Most of those who have written about grieving, beginning with Freud on the necessity of "decathexis,"[8] or emotional separation, tell us that we need to relinquish virtually all our ties to the deceased in order to avoid a morbid longing for their return, preoccupation with the past or with the introjected memory of the dead, or identification with the dead to the detriment of our individuality. I agree that we must overcome or avoid static, fixed, lifeless, preoccupying, or obsessive connections with the deceased if we are to progress as we grieve. The traditional view includes, quite possibly as its core, the assertion that we need to resist the temptations of the potentially paralyzing extreme grief emotion that entails unrelenting and preoccupying longing for the impossible return of the deceased (see Chapter 2). As Kathryn keeps her promise to Mark, she firmly resolves not to allow longing for his return to consume her. Despite Sheila's unanticipated death when their reconciliation had just begun, Colleen, too, recognizes that longing for her daughter's return is futile. Others, however, might dwell in extreme grief, even with its attendant pain and anguish, as the only way they can imagine to keep their love for the deceased alive.

We cannot remain dependent on or under the destructively controlling influence of the deceased. Dependence and possessiveness (including attempts to control or manipulate, even abusively) compromise, undermine, or stifle the full development of our personal subjectivity and individuality. Sometimes it may take the shock of death to reveal when such predeath morbidity is part of our loving relationships. Fortunately, neither Kathryn nor Colleen was dependent on or controlled by Mark or Sheila. Breaking the chains of our dependence on or control by others can be very liberating, and our doing so as survivors constitutes an insistence that the deceased "let go" of us.

When we are bereaved, some of us may become "stuck" or fixed in relation to the deceased in other ways. When we lack strong identities of our own, we sometimes identify excessively with the deceased as we either take on the characteristics of the illness or the condition that led to the death or make ourselves so much like the deceased that we lose our own identities and compromise our own personal development. Neither Kathryn nor Colleen has such difficulty.

Others of us become caught up in "unfinished business" with the deceased as we become preoccupied, frozen, and at a loss as to how to resolve the lingering tensions between us. We may feel an all-consuming anger or hatred in response to abuse or other harm we suffered at the hands of the deceased or an equally consuming guilt over having ourselves abused, harmed, or failed the deceased. Some mourners long for the return of the deceased as the only way they can imagine to address such unfinished business.

It is not only positive ties in our love relationships that can bind us to the deceased in extreme grief. Colleen's issues of guilt and anger, forgiveness and self-forgiveness in her unhappy relationship with Sheila could stall her grieving. Her failed attempts to possess Sheila and keep her dependent haunt her. Fortunately, she finds information gathering and prayer to be effective ways to address her unfinished business.

Negative legacies in love relationships can undermine us as we struggle to relearn our worlds and our selves or hold us in unresolved tensions. When we do not understand how constructive and life-affirming continued loving of the deceased is possible and want desperately to keep love alive or to maintain our relationship with the deceased in some form, we may linger in the emotion grief or otherwise cling to the deceased in morbid and destructive ways.

Disentangling ourselves from the paralyzing or otherwise lingering destructive effects and influences of relationships does not require that we sever all our ties to the deceased. The only additional "letting go" that is required of us is precisely that required in our loving relationships when the others are present, fully alive, and respected as individuals in their own right—that we relinquish any fixed expectations and cultivate tolerance for, expectation of, and excitement in the changing face, influence, and inspiration of the other. As we learn how to love in absence after death, we may recover a vital, nondependent, nonpossessive connection with the deceased that we knew prior to the death, or we may become capable of such letting go for the first time if the relationship was unhealthy in its possessiveness prior to the death. Kathryn learned well of such letting go with Mark while he was alive. Colleen was just beginning to learn of it when Sheila died unexpectedly and tragically. Part of Colleen's grieving as she wrestles with forgiveness and self-forgiveness involves learning more fully of such letting go. If we can achieve a dynamic, life-affirming, life-promoting, and enriching relationship with the deceased, we will not need to let go entirely, and we will avoid morbidity.

We Continue to Love and Cherish the Stories of Lives Now Ended

Though our bonding with one another has its source in physical interaction, our mature attachments transcend such concrete beginnings. Thus, we continue our connections with others even when we are separated from them while they are alive. Such connections are much more abstract, as we discover, appreciate, and allow ourselves to be motivated by the values and meanings embodied in the lives of the others and in our interactions with them. When others die, we experience the pain of loss of their physical presence. However, death does not cancel their lives, though they end physically. Kathryn and especially Colleen rightly resist the advice of those who urge them to go on as if Mark and Sheila had never lived. That would be impossible and profoundly disorienting for them. The reality within which Kathryn and Colleen must reorient themselves is one in which Mark and Sheila changed irreversibly their worlds and their lives. Moreover, they have not lost the value and meaning of Mark's and Sheila's lives. Though their lives have ended, their survivors can continue to appreciate those values and meanings, which remain untouched by temporal events. Whether or not there is life after death, or a literal immortality, as Colleen believes, each of us attains what Robert Lifton calls our "symbolic immortality."[9] As we acknowledge and learn to live with the values and meanings of the lives now ended, we come to know and appreciate the lingering, symbolically immortal aspects of those lives. As we do so, we realize the eternal value of those lives.

What might our continued, dynamic, loving connection with the deceased be like? The metaphor of the continuation of the dance even as the partners part suggests that the attentiveness and responsiveness involved might be like reading a dance partner. To extend and deepen our understanding of such a connection, I suggest that we think of our continuing to love the deceased as being like reading, interpreting, and living in dynamic interaction with the fully developed stories of their lives. As we come to know and love others, we come to know and cherish the stories of the lives they live, as Kathryn and Colleen came to know and cherish the stories of Mark and Sheila. If we have known and loved well (as Kathryn and Colleen have), the stories become interwoven with the fabric of the stories of our lives. Kathryn recalls and appreciates the vivid positive legacy Mark left her. Colleen struggles with the ambivalence in her relationship with Sheila and the often painful legacy of her life. As we relearn our relationship with the deceased, we continue the interweaving process. In all of our relationships we have unique and privileged access to parts of the full stories of others' lives. Our knowledge and love of the stories remain after the loss of the presence of the deceased. Some stories are far shorter than others, but even the life of an infant, a newborn, a stillborn, or a miscarried child is a life with a history that we can find meaningful and in which we have typically invested much hope. There is, consequently, a story to be told, heard, and remembered, even in such seemingly limiting cases. As survivors, we continue to love the deceased dynamically as we grow and develop understanding and appreciation of the stories in their own right and of their significance for our living as survivors.

Kathryn continues to weave the predominantly positive legacy of Mark's life into the web of her life after his death. She seeks ways to allow that legacy to shape the remaining years of her life and to share it with Josh and Sarah. Similarly, Colleen continues to weave Sheila's complex (and potentially negative) legacy into the web of her life. She struggles to retain and cherish what is good and what she can learn from Sheila and her past relationship with her and to free herself from the possibly crippling effects of the unfinished business of anger and guilt.

As with any good stories, but especially with the intricate stories of human biography, if we read them but once we fail to capture the richness and fullness of the tales. As we review and retell stories repeatedly, they return ever new and unexpected rewards each time. We can always reinterpret the stories, and as we do so, we can deepen our appreciation of the values and meanings they reveal. We cannot completely and definitively interpret stories in principle, since each reading comes at a different point in our lives, and we bring changing background experiences, perspectives, interests, needs, and desires to the interpretive context. As with any good stories, but again especially with the stories of a loved one's life, we can return to the stories deliberately for specific purposes (to refresh our memory or understanding or to seek new understanding) or as events in our lives remind us of them and of their continuing importance to us.

Kathryn's reversions to the story of Mark's life in private and her retellings of it with Sarah and Josh at Thanksgiving and on Mark's birthday yield new rewards for all. The freshness of the story each time and its power to affect them continually amaze her. Each year the children are older, ask different questions, want to know different details, laugh and cry at different points, and talk differently of the retelling in the days and weeks that follow. Mark is most certainly neither forgotten nor frozen in photographic images. Rather, he remains a living presence in his children's lives as they grow and develop and meet the challenges of relearning their worlds in their father's absence. Kathryn, too, reaches new points in her personal development and appreciates different aspects of the story each time she revisits it. Early reversions to it ground her growing self-understanding, and later ones refresh her memory and rekindle cherished inspiration.

Colleen at first desperately seeks to know more of the details of Sheila's life that were lost to her because of their estrangement. As she learns more, she constantly reinterprets the story. She is deeply touched by those who generously share what they remember, reveal aspects of Sheila's life and character that were unknown to her, tell her what Sheila cared about (including interests she shared with her mother), and offer their perspectives on the values and meanings of Sheila's life. Colleen reinterprets Sheila's life story as she learns new details, comes to different points in her own growing self-understanding, and sees her relationship with Sheila in new light. She is also returned to the story repeatedly by the anger and guilt that weigh so heavily on her; that is, she is drawn to it by her need to resolve lingering tensions in her relationship with Sheila.

Rarely are we alone in knowing and loving the stories of the lives of others. When others die, we can, and often want to, share stories with others who can fill in for us additional chapters of the narratives from their perspectives. Both confirmation of and discontinuity with our own interpretations of the stories are possible; in exchange with others, we can deepen and enhance indefinitely our understanding and appreciation of the fullness and the lasting value of the stories. As we together share and cherish the stories of lives now ended, we add immeasurably to both our individual and our community lives.

Not only did Kathryn's remarkable invitation to others to remember him move Mark profoundly before he died, but Kathryn, Josh, and Sarah benefit in their grief as they share memories and stories, many of which otherwise might have remained unknown to them. The generosity of others provides them with a much richer legacy of Mark's life to treasure in the coming years. Their open and repeated recounting of the stories enriches their individual lives and enhances the bonds between them. Colleen, too, benefits from others' sharing their knowledge and interpretations of the details of Sheila's life, most of which she would have otherwise never known. What they have to tell helps her sort more effectively the mixed legacy of Sheila's life. It pains her to realize that most of her family and friends are either unwilling or unable to join in remembering and talking about the life she finds too precious to forget.

In our lifetimes we learn many stories, but we hold close to very few, finding in them special significance and staying power as they speak to what matters most to us. While it would be obsessive for us to become entirely absorbed and preoccupied by but one story, we can give a single story considerably more attention and treasure it over the years, returning to it frequently, without becoming obsessive. It is important for us to put down the story of the life of deceased and attend to other stories, to become involved in life with our fellow survivors. But it is also important for us to continue to love the story, hold it dear and cherish it, keep it available, recognize its lasting value, and, in returning to it, be absorbed in loving it for its sustaining freshness and renewing vitality. Our ongoing dynamic interaction with the stories of loved ones' lives can return rewards comparable to those found in a lifelong interaction with the greatest texts ever written. If this metaphor has any power whatever, it undercuts the traditional view's insistence that we must relinquish all ties with the deceased, that is, that our letting go must be complete.

We can find much that interests us in the stories of those who have died. As we can interact with and love others in many ways while they live, so, too, can we continue to interact with and love the stories of their lives in many ways in their absence. Kierkegaard tells us that there are three basic ways of living in the world, or caring: the aesthetic, the ethical, and the religious.[10] In the first, the *aesthetic*, we live and interact with others because we find them interesting. Though the texts of the lives of the deceased are finished, we can still explore them endlessly and take an infinite interest in them as objects of our fascination, just as we can find any human life far more interesting than the story of any thing. We may plumb the aesthetic values and meanings of the lives of the deceased alone or with others. As we do so, the stories we treasure may move us to laughter or tears. At times the stories may simply delight or bring us joy as we escape into pleasant memories of them; at others they may arouse our curiosity, provoke us to reflect and examine ourselves deeply, inspire us to appreciate mystery, remind us of the fragility and wonder of life itself, or evoke in us a sense of tragedy.

Kathryn appreciates Mark in memory both alone and with her children. Sometimes she laughs; at other times she cries. Inviting friends and family to write appreciations before Mark died in part satisfied her curiosity about aspects of his life that were unknown to her. Sessions with their mother amply reward Sarah's and Josh's curiosity about their father, who died when they were so young. Kathryn marvels at how much she learns about herself as she remembers Mark. Always she appreciates the unfathomable mystery of a life lived by another, the fragile but nevertheless precious character of her too few years with Mark, and the poignant tragedy of the death of one so young and filled with promise.

Colleen appreciates Sheila in memory while alone, in her interviews with Sheila's West Coast friends, and in dialogue with God. Tears predominate over laughter, though there is some of the latter. The interviews and journal keeping satisfy her curiosity about the lost years. She also learns much about herself as she remembers. The intricacies of human relationship and the interconnectedness of things prove fascinating mysteries as they become apparent in her reversions to Sheila's life. She recognizes only too well how fragile yet wonderful the life of another is and also knows the poignant tragedy of the death of one so young and filled with promise.

We can also be moved to "do the right thing" by the stories of those who have died. In the second of Kierkegaard's ways of caring, the *ethical*, we live or interact with others in a way that moves us to live by moral principles or to take on responsibility. While there is room for us to mourn as a way of performing a duty to the dead, there is a danger of morbidity in this if we carry it beyond reasonable

limits, or if we act on promises or feelings of responsibility or loyalty to the deceased that require that we not love again or restrict
arbitrarily our involvements in the world in which we survive and
they do not. It is best that we surmount such negative legacies of
control from beyond the grave. However, we can also commit ourselves to the deceased to carry on in their absence, to return to fully
involved caring in the world. Obligations to the dead need not entail
excessive devotion, adoration, or self-sacrifice from us. Rather, our
lives can be shaped at least in part by feelings of responsibility to the
deceased or to the commitments that we shared and undertook with
them. There need be no more morbidity in our sustaining covenants
with the dead than in our doing so with the living.

Kathryn made no destructive or constricting promises to Mark
that hinder her as she relearns her world and transforms herself after his death. In fact, her promise to him not to allow grief to overcome her motivates her to do these things and to learn life-affirming
ways of loving him in his absence. She neither devotes herself to
nor adores him excessively. As she allows herself to be influenced
by Mark in his absence, she makes no inappropriate self-sacrifice;
quite the opposite. As she helps Sarah and Josh remember and know
him as a real person, she both keeps a promise to Mark and enriches
all their lives. As she "consults" Mark at points of key decision,
such as whether to pursue her career interests and to remarry, she
constructively sustains her covenants with Mark and remains faithful to the best of the love they knew when he was alive.

Colleen struggles to surmount the continuing effects of the negative legacy of (as she sees it) her having failed Sheila after the divorce. She acknowledges her smothering, protecting, and controlling,
sees them as ethically problematic, and seeks forgiveness from
Sheila, God, and herself. While she made no destructive promises to
Sheila and is not controlled by her from beyond the grave, her own
"failures" pain her, and she resists their preoccupying her. She resolves to learn from her mistakes and make constructive changes in
her life and ways of interacting with others. She is determined that
such changes be a positive legacy of her relationship with Sheila.

Last, *we can be moved spiritually and take self-transforming
inspiration from the stories of those who have died.* In the third of
Kierkegaard's ways of caring, the *religious,* we live or interact with
others in full appreciation of human limitation and fallibility and in
recognition of the transcending power of the eternal. We stand before the mystery, presence, and transcendence of another in wonder
and awe. As survivors, we understand and appreciate the eternal

value of the life now ended, for the value and meaning that were in it are untouched by the death. We recognize the indelible imprint, the irreplaceable uniqueness, of the life of the deceased and the love and caring manifest within it. In what Martin Buber called the "I-Thou" relationship,[11] we stand in genuine dialogue with a sense of the privilege of knowing the independent reality of the other and being transformed by the exchange. As we continue to love the deceased, we retain and increase our appreciation of the gift that was his or her life. We can remain in such dialogue if we continue to explore and allow ourselves to be affected by that gift of the other life. In turn, as we recognize the gift-like character of the life of the deceased, we may wonder at the mysteries of the universe itself within which such gifts are provided through no dessert or effort on our part. We then experience in awe and reverence, ponder in meditation or reflection, and interact in prayer with, the divine. We experience its mysteries as grounding and encompassing our relationship with the deceased. In prayers of grace we express appreciation for the gift. In prayers of confession we seek forgiveness. In prayers of supplication we seek to renew hope, motivation, resolve, and dedication in continuing relationship with the deceased.

The freshness and fullness of Mark's continuing presence in her life amazes Kathryn as she "consults" him and imagines what he might have recommended in unprecedented situations. Reversions to the story of his life prompt new insights into his character and provoke novel responses. Death does not cancel the values and meanings of Mark's life. She realizes how she is indelibly different for having known him. The extent of his inspiration is greater than she comprehends. By the time she marries Jim, she appreciates how irreplaceable Mark is. She is grateful for her having known and been transformed in the knowing, and so is Jim. Together, they and the children treasure the gift of Mark's life. This is especially so in the "remember-when" sessions with Sarah and Josh. In prayer she gives thanks and prays for sustained hope and sense of purpose in going on without Mark.

Colleen, unfortunately, realizes and appreciates very late how Sheila, in her own person and as the subject at the center of her own world of experience, transcends her smothering and controlling grasp. She sees how her crushing possessiveness drove Sheila away and deprived her of opportunities to know Sheila better, love her more gently and respectfully, and possibly be loved by her in return. She feels the pain of not having had the gift of the lost years. Her efforts to reconstruct them, though successful, provide but a glimpse of the fullness of the life she might have known better. Her willingness to explore and be affected by the gift of that life, painful though it is, contributes to her self-understanding and self-transformation. She prays for Sheila's soul for having taken her own life. She gives thanks for the privilege of knowing Sheila and for what she continues to learn from having known her. She seeks forgiveness from God, perhaps as a condition for granting it to herself. Last, she prays for new understanding of her grief and the meaning of life and in the hope of one day being reunited with Sheila.

We Still Care About What Those Who Died Cared About

What place might continued loving of the dead hold in our lives as survivors as we redefine our personal identities? In loving others, we care about what they care about, share their concerns and values. In some cases we do this only because they care, and we recognize how that caring is integral to their flourishing. We care for their sake. In other cases, we make their cares genuinely our own as we appropriate the cares and values into our own identities and ways of living in the world. The cares then come to function for us as what Kierkegaard called "subjective truths";[12] that is, they give meaning and direction to our lives as survivors. We value the objects of care for their own sake and not merely for their having held such a prominent place in the lives of those we cared about and loved. As we survive, we can thrive in an enjoyment and an appreciation of and a heightened sensitivity to life that derives from our having known and loved the deceased. We can sense that we walk in the world as their representatives as they may have wished nothing more than that we would live fully and richly in their absence. As we appropriate some of their values and cares, we can respond inventively to the loss and live productively in memory of those who have contributed much to our lives. As we continue, deepen, and sometimes transform our caring about what they cared about, we can pay homage to their memory. As we care about what they cared about, we continue to love them. Moreover, our love can encompass our gratitude for their having helped us to become the kind of persons who care in such ways. We need not be dependent or self-effacing as we identify with the dead and appreciate their contributions to our identities.

Our relearning of our relationships with the deceased contributes to the emergence of our new personal identities and the achievement of a new wholeness in our current living, personal history, and connection to larger wholes. We reweave into newly integrated patterns of our current living threads of caring that first were woven into the webs of our lives while the deceased lived. We reintegrate the values and meanings of the stories of the lives now ended into our own life stories as we reinterpret our past life with the deceased, alter the ways we live in the present, and project new hopes and purposes into the future. And we join our changed connections with the deceased to our modified connections with our family, friends, the larger community, God, and life projects as we again connect meaningfully with self-transcending wholes. As we find or achieve wholeness in each of these ways, we constructively identify with the deceased; that is, we define who we are in terms of our continuing relationships with them in their absence. We reintegrate ouselves as we find new places for love of the deceased in our lives.

Kathryn interacts with Mark in her daily life as she consults at the cemetery, twirls her wedding ring, and prays. He is present in memory and inspiration as she reshapes her daily routine, raises their children, and makes major decisions. As her life story takes a new course with her career development and, later, her remarriage, she carries Mark's story with her and draws inspiration from it. The remember-when sessions with the children support both her own reintegration of his story into her own life and the continuing integration of it into Josh's and Sarah's lives. Though she derives the greatest satisfaction from the children, her career, and her new husband, Jim, she still connects meaningfully with Mark. She is grateful that her relationship with Mark will always be part of who she has been, who she is, and who she becomes.

Colleen interacts with Sheila in her daily life in prayer, in her continuing interests in literature, theater, and the environment, and in her struggles with guilt, anger, forgiveness, and self-forgiveness. Her investigation into the lost years supports her as she reinterprets her past as wife and mother. It motivates her to examine herself and to learn from her mistakes, and it instills a hope that she will eventually learn to carry with her and to cherish the story of Sheila's life without the pain it currently arouses. She grows confident that she can become a different and better person for having known and loved her daughter. As she works through her unfinished business and more fully appreciates Sheila as a person in her own right, Colleen connects lovingly with her daughter as she never did while she lived.

Loving the dead is compatible with our forming new relationships, though it can complicate it. We can enter a new relationship in a way that no more abandons or betrays the deceased than when we add friends to our lives. Indeed, it may accord with the fondest wishes of the deceased. Where cultures define, and we experience, some relationships, such as marriage, as more exclusive, we must abandon the exclusivity (not the deceased or the continued loving) if we choose to form a new relationship.

Kathryn and Jim form a new marital bond and yet find room for continuing relationships with Mark and with Jim's first wife. Each appreciates how the other is who she or he is (and lovable in being so) by virtue of the earlier relationship. Each respects the other's need to maintain connection to the deceased and is sensitive to the other as he or she does so primarily in private. Jim especially appreciates the importance of Kathryn's keeping Mark's story alive for Josh and Sarah as they grow and develop. Complications could have arisen had either been less flexible in defining their new relationship or intolerant of the continuing connections with those who died.

Advantages of the Idea of Relearning Our Relationships with the Deceased

The Idea Provides Understanding

Those of us who desire it can find a dynamic, life-affirming, life-promoting, enriching, and, most often, loving connection with those who have died. We can reintegrate our relationships with the deceased into a new personal wholeness in all the ways that I discussed in Chapter 5: We can incorporate caring about the deceased as a person in his or her own right, and caring about what the deceased cared about, into our newly coherent daily lives. We can reinterpret and reshape our life stories as we revert to, appreciate the values of, reinterpret the meanings of, accept the influence of, and take inspiration from the stories of, those we have cared about and loved. As we maintain our relationships, we can derive meaning and purpose from an abiding self-transcending connection.

This understanding allows us to reinterpret several aspects of our experiences as survivors. Part of what we do when we relearn the world is learn how to sustain a loving connection with the dead or disentangle ourselves from the destructive negative legacies of our unhappy but still binding relationships. We must relinquish our concrete loving of the presence of those we have cared about and replace it with abstract loving in separation; our yearning and searching reflect the pain of letting go of the physical attachment. That we

must experience this pain does not mean that we must let go entirely of all attachment to the deceased. Finding a way to love without physical presence can help us move from dwelling in this pain
to carrying it as a far less pervasive aspect of our lives. We must
overcome the emotionally crippling effects of dependence, possessiveness, and other dysfunctional aspects of our relationships if we
are to progress as we grieve and make the transition to loving in
separation (or, in some cases, to disentangle altogether).

When we are bereaved, we may fear both letting go of those
who have died and losing ourselves in the past if we do not let go.
Completely severing our relationships with the dead is unneces-
sary, though the fixity of, for example, dependence or possessiveness is undesirable. As we come to understand the life-affirming
potential of loving in separation, we can overcome our fear of morbidity, and our common, and often fervent, desire to remain linked
to the dead can be validated.

The Idea Promotes Respect for Individuality

No two of our relationships are identical. We communicate in distinct ways; cooperate and interact distinctively in daily life; share
unique memories, present experiences, hopes, and aspirations; interweave our life histories in idiosyncratic ways; develop personal
understandings of ourselves and others; realize values and find
meanings unique to the relationships; experience ambivalence; and
accumulate personal unfinished business. In all of these ways, and
in others, the deceased, when alive, found distinctive places in our
daily life patterns, personal life histories, and sense of connectedness. Respect for our individuality when we grieve requires that
others appreciate the significance of each of these aspects of our
relationship with the deceased as it is affected by the death.

No two of us relearn our relationship with the deceased by
meeting identical challenges. Reintegration of our relationships
within our present living, in understanding of our individual autobiographies, and in our new patterns of self-transcending connection
demands different things of each of us. Each of us takes a distinctive
course, and, as we do so, the deceased finds a unique place in each of
our lives as our losses and grieving transform them.

The Idea Addresses Our Helplessness

As I first noted in Chapter 2, extreme grief can cripple and even
paralyze us. In it we experience the futility of our desire to have the

person we loved (or, for that matter, hated) returned in living presence. Dwelling in extreme grief makes us helpless and powerless. Still, some of us remain in extreme grief in part out of fear that if we let go of the desire for the deceased's physical return, that will end our loving. It is possible to interact meaningfully with the deceased in their absence, love them, have and hold them dear, without dwelling in extreme grief. Understanding this can help us overcome the fear of relinquishing our desire for the return of the deceased that can hold us in the emotion grief and free us actively to relearn ourselves and our worlds.

We can continue to "have" what we have "lost," that is, a continuing, albeit transformed, love for the deceased. We have not truly lost our years of living with the deceased or our memories. Nor have we lost the influences, the inspirations, the values, and the meanings embodied in their lives. We can actively incorporate these into new patterns of living that include transformed but abiding relationships with those we have cared about and loved. This understanding can motivate and support our return to dynamic, life-affirming living in which the gift of the life of the deceased continues to give and to be appreciated by us.

The Idea Provides Guidance for Caregivers

As caregivers, we can be with the bereaved as they experience and express the anguish of letting go of the concrete reality of the dead. We can listen patiently and understandingly to the pain at the loss of presence, offer comfort and support and give it when it is welcomed. But we need not, and indeed should not, encourage complete letting go of the deceased. We can reassure the bereaved that the desire for a continuing relationship with the deceased is normal and not necessarily, or even usually, morbid. We can support and nurture their potential for continued, albeit transformed, loving of the deceased by sharing memories and stories of our own as they are available.

We can support and encourage others as they grieve to remember and explore the narrative of the life now ended for its sustaining value and meaning. Here we can encourage retelling of the stories of the lives lived and treasured. Retelling makes the lives real and freshens and enlivens memory. We can encourage retelling during the funeral period. We can encourage grieving persons to establish times and places to revisit the story, such as birthdays, anniversaries, or holidays, in a quiet place at home, at a place of worship, or at a graveside. We can encourage them to keep a diary or journal as a means of accumulating a fuller record of cherished memories.

We can support them as they record their and others' memories on audio or videotape, or we can encourage them to write pieces about their most unforgettable experiences with the deceased.

We can promote and encourage grieving persons to fill in details of the lives as they may be available from diverse sources. When the death is anticipated, we can encourage life review with those who are dying before death comes. We can encourage those who grieve to invite others to share details of the stories during visitation, at funerals or memorial services, or later. Many who grieve long for the reassurance this provides that others, too, cared for the deceased. We can encourage them to seek out and informally interview persons to draw from them aspects of the lives of the deceased that they may not know, as Colleen did. We can encourage them to solicit letters or stories from others, as Kathryn did, or to engage in the equivalent of genealogical research. We can encourage them to establish occasions for sharing the story, for example, at anniversary, birthday, or holiday gatherings.

We can encourage those who grieve to continue to explore the diverse aesthetic, ethical, and religious meanings, influences, and inspirations embodied in the stories of the lives now ended. We can encourage them to extend diary writing or journal keeping beyond simple record keeping to include reflections on why the lives of the deceased are so memorable, what they cherish in them, or how they are better for having known the deceased. In an aesthetic way of caring, we can encourage them to appreciate the interest of the story, the joys, delight, laughter, tears, and fascination it arouses in them and its provocative, curious, mysterious, and perhaps even tragic aspects.

Caring in an ethical framework, we can encourage those who grieve to appreciate the moral dimension and significance of the stories. We can explore with them ways of meeting any responsibilities they feel they now have because they knew the deceased. We can support them as they mull over how to find ways of going on that reflect commitments inspired by, values instilled by, or promises and covenants entered into with the deceased. We can support them as they find new resolve and give new direction to their lives in ways that the deceased inspired.

Last, to demonstrate our caring in a religious context, we can encourage those who grieve to appreciate the spiritual and religious dimensions of the stories now ended, including the transcendence of others, the wonder and awe of standing before the independent reality of the deceased, and the challenges that the deceased's separate lives continue to present to those who survive them. We can encourage them to reflect on the abiding meaning of the lives now ended, which are not canceled by death. We can invite them to consider how they may continue in dialogue with the deceased, how they may continue to be affected by the gift of knowing them. We can support them as they struggle to forgive the deceased for their limitations and fallibility. We can encourage prayers of grace, in which they express gratitude for the privilege of knowing and being a part of the stories; prayers of confession, in which they seek self-forgiveness for what they perceive to be failings in interaction with the deceased; and prayers of supplication, in which they seek to arouse a renewal of hope, motivation, resolve, and rededication in terms of a continuing loving relationship with the deceased.

As caregivers, we can help those who grieve to discern ways in which they can continue to care about what those who died cared about. We can support them in sustaining dynamic, nonobsessive loving connectedness with the deceased by living in terms of those cares. We can also support them as they attempt to disentangle themselves from any destructive, fixating, and dysfunctional connections that may remain. We can use concrete objects and mementos to help them make the transition from concrete relation in presence to abstract relation in absence. We can relieve their guilt over new involvements in projects or relationships by urging them to explore whether the deceased's love for them included a desire that they continue to live fully and to flourish. We can help survivors discern what has not been lost of the value and meaning of the lives of those who have died and continue to treasure the gifts of the lives of the deceased that are still theirs. We can motivate them actively to relearn their worlds and to let go of extreme grief emotion by bringing this end into view—the goal of recovering the fruits of the lives now ended.

Notes

1. C. S. Lewis, *A Grief Observed* (New York: Bantam Books, 1976), pp. 58–59.

2. Recall the discussion in Chapter 5 of grieving as a struggle to transcend suffering and to reestablish wholeness in our selves.

3. Lewis, *A Grief*, p. 52.

4. Ibid., p. 59.

5. Alan Watts, *The Wisdom of Insecurity* (New York: Random House, 1968), p. 32.

6. Ibid., p. 24.

7. Lewis, *A Grief*, p. 77.

8. Sigmund Freud, *Totem and Taboo* in *Standard Edition of the Complete Psychological Works of Sigmund Freud*, vol. 13 (London: Hogarth Press, 1955). See Dennis Klass, "John Bowlby's Model of Grief and the Problem of Identification," Appendix 2, in *Parental Grief: Solace and Resolution* (New York: Springer Publishing Company, 1988), pp. 193–214, for a detailed discussion of the history of thinking along these lines.

9. Robert Lifton, *The Broken Connection* (New York: Basic Books, 1983).

10. Soren Kierkegaard, *Stages on Life's Way*, trans. Walter Lowrie (Princeton, N.J.: Princeton University Press, 1940).

11. Martin Buber, *I and Thou*, trans. Walter Kaufmann (New York: Charles Scribner's Sons, 1970).

12. Kierkegaard, *Stages on Life's Way*.

Index

Absence, love in, l–liv, 174–91
Accessibility
  of ideas of grieving, 11–12
  of medical views, 45
  of the relearning view, 122
  of stage/phase views, 45
  of task-based views, 56
Activity
  in grieving, xxx–xxxvi, 33, 41–42, 47–61, 122
  meaning in, 69–71
Achievement values
  definition, 70
  discussion, 69–71
Aesthetic caring, 181–82, 190
Ambivalence, 80–82, 115, 136–37, 176–78
Amelioration of distress and anguish, 144–45, 152–56
Analogies. *See also* Web metaphor for personal integrity; Web of webs metaphor for family and community
  inadequate, 44–47, 157–58
  usefulness, 12, 24 *n.* 5
Anger, 42–43, 80–84, 115, 118, 169, 177–80, 186

Anguish, 144–45, 152–56, 170–74. *See also* Grief—the emotion, extreme; Helplessness
Anticipated death. *See* Kathryn; Louise; Martin
Anticipatory grief, liv
Assumptions, xlii, 107–8. *See also* Expectations
Assumptive world, loss of, xlii–xliii
Atomistic view of selves, 157–58
Attachment, 37, 48. *See also* Connections; Longing; Love

Behavioral coping. *See* Coping with loss, behavioral
Beliefs
  challenged in bereavement, 55, 89, 92, 116, 119
  disbelief, 42
  faith, 14, 23, 53, 72–73, 89–91, 96, 119–21, 151–52, 154
  in grief—the emotion, 34–36
  reviewed in coping, 96, 121, 125–26. *See also* Coping with loss, intellectual/spiritual
  about what happened, 115

CPSIA information can be obtained
at www.ICGtesting.com
Printed in the USA
BVHW012026061022
648867BV00011B/140